Gut Reactions

Understanding Symptoms of the Digestive Tract

W. Grant Thompson, M.D.

Professor of Medicine
Chief, Division of Gastroenterology
and Digestive Diseases Research Unit
Ottawa Civic Hospital
and University of Ottawa
Ottawa, Ontario, Canada

Plenum Press • New York and London

Library of Congress Cataloging in Publication Data

Thompson, W. Grant.
    Gut reactions: understanding symptoms of the digestive tract / W. Grant Thompson.
        p.   cm.
    Bibliography: p.
    Includes index.
    ISBN 0-306-43303-6
    1. Irritable colon. 2. Gastrointestinal system—Diseases. 3. Symptomatology. I.
Title.
RC862.I77T46   1989   89-16048
616.3'42—dc20   CIP

First Printing—August 1989
Second Printing—April 1990

The treatments outlined in this volume are intended to serve
only as examples. You should consult your personal physician
before beginning any medical treatment regimen.

TO SUE

Preface

All of us have gut reactions. We often respond to strong emotion or changes in circumstances with such digestive symptoms as nausea, heartburn, abdominal discomfort, or altered bowel habit. Travel, examinations, public speaking, and dietary indiscretions are familiar provocations. No serious disease accounts for these reactions, which appear to be the way the gut responds, or is perceived to respond, to its owner's physical and psychosocial environment. Although most people consider them part of life, for others the symptoms may be sufficiently frequent, troublesome, and inexplicable that they are said to have an irritable gut. Thus, the various gut reactions, if frequent and troublesome, are syndromes of the irritable gut. It seems that at least one third of people suffer with one or more of the irritable gut syndromes that are discussed in this book. Many of these sufferers seek medical care, undergo many tests, and receive treatments that are costly and not often effective.

There is a need to demystify the irritable gut or at least make the sufferer more comfortable in contemplating his gut reactions. The truth is, we do not understand them very well. Several facts do stand out. The reactions are very common and affect people most of their lives. They are benign, that is, they do not lead to any serious diseases, nor is there any structural or anatomical abnormality to explain them. They seem to be due to altered physiology (function) or at least to altered perception of physiology. Lastly, there is no reliable cure.

Thus, this book is written for patients, their relatives, and those nurses, physicians, and allied health workers who may wish to understand digestive symptoms better. There are no tests or x-rays that will identify these gut reactions, but they are clearly recognizable from their symptoms and are not just what is left when organic disease is excluded through many tests. The commonness of these disorders and their positive diagnosis may be comforting to sufferers. It is reassuring for an individual to know that his or her irritable gut is a real entity experienced by other people, and that it does not indicate cancer or other mortal illness.

So my purpose in this book is to improve the understanding of gut reactions, because I believe the reader's comprehension and reassurance that no serious disease exists is most important and, in many cases, the only treatment. Certainly, attention to emotional stress, life-style, and diet may help as well. Furthermore, it is my purpose to dissuade us all, sufferers, physicians and others, from the costly and sometimes harmful notions that many tests are necessary and that there must be a drug to make the patient better. Interpretation of symptoms is the only reliable test, and drugs, even if they seem to help in the short term, are seldom a sensible life time solution.

Part 1 reviews the anatomy and physiology for nonmedical readers, then the definitions of bowel habit and the various irritable gut syndromes. A discussion of the prevalence of these disorders in the community and their considerable cost follows next. Since lack of dietary fiber and emotion are recurring themes thought to be very important in the irritable gut, they are assigned a chapter each.

In Part 2, ten chapters describe the various syndromes of the irritable gut. Gut reactions appear to result from abnormal function or abnormal perception of function at all levels of the gut. Although we know that symptoms are seated in the esophagus, stomach, small or large intestine, we know little about their genesis. No one sufferer will have all of these syndromes, but many will have more than one. Thus, an understanding of the whole picture may help the sufferer cope with his or her own gut reactions. Certainly the key chapter in this section is "The Irritable Bowel," Chapter 13.

The five chapters in Part 3 discuss topics that are important to those patients with gut reactions. Diverticula occur in half the population by age 60. It is a popular misconception that the diverticula themselves cause symptoms. They don't, but an irritable bowel may be coincidentally present. Laxatives and other drugs cause many gut symptoms and the sufferer should recognize these. Chapter 21, "Clinical Trials and the Placebo Response," demonstrates that most drugs used for gut reactions have very little scientific justification. We accept too easily the notion that there must be a drug out there that will help. In this context, an understanding of the placebo response is a fundamental issue. The final chapter describes some of the tests irritable gut patients commonly undergo. Most gut reactions reported to a physician require an x-ray, an endoscopy, or a stool collection, and it is helpful if the sufferer knows what to expect.

I hope that the reader will recognize gut reactions as important medical problems, not only for the discomfort and worry they engender but also for their great prevalence and the cost of their investigation and treatment. As threats to humanity, they cannot claim the profile of cancer or heart disease, but they do cause discomfort in many people and can divert resources from the detection and care of more serious diseases. On these grounds, research into how the gut functions and how we perceive its function is important. Meanwhile, we can only combine what few facts we have about gut reactions with common sense, and resolve that we will not permit our zeal for tests and cure to exceed reason or to do harm.

The bibliography is brief and confined to key or review articles that should satisfy the need of most readers to seek out the original references. Much of the material prior to 1979 is referenced in my previous book, *The Irritable Gut*. Lest one think I refer excessively to my own work, it should be clear that most original references for the material in this book are contained therein.

Gut reactions are part of the human condition. The classical references and quotes from the old medical literature serve, I hope, to emphasize the timeless humanity of these disorders. Although they are said to be products of Western civilization, I believe all mankind is liable. Gut reactions occasionally inspire humor, for the gut has always been a source of mirth. Those sufferers who regard their symptoms very seriously should not be offended by this, for with humor comes recognition of the human condition, and from thence compassion.

                                                            W. Grant Thompson
Mont Tremblant, Quebec

Acknowledgments

This book owes much to my recently deceased parents, George and Florence Thompson, who oversaw my education and insisted that my experience should be as broad as possible. Of course, the completion of the book would have been impossible without the support of my wife, Sue, who helped edit the manuscript, and the good-humored patience of my children, Julie, Jennifer, and Eric. Jennifer prepared the Index.

Another key person is Helen Kierczak, whose Tandy word processor actually created the manuscript, and who, when I despaired of completion, always had a cheerful word of encouragement. James Harbinson's illustrations speak for themselves.

The x-rays that are in the book are due to the courtesy of Dr. Hardy Tao, Department of Radiology, Ottawa Civic Hospital. Photographs were taken by Stuart Joyce and Tom Devecseri of the Civic Hospital's Audio Visual Department.

The ideas for this book have developed over 20 years. During that period I have been privileged to discuss the irritable gut with many colleagues from several countries. Special mention is due to Dr. K. W. Heaton of Bristol, England, and Dr. D. A. Drossman of Chapel Hill, North Carolina. The irritable gut has made us good friends. I cannot forget the support and encouragement of many colleagues at the University of Ottawa—Dean Gilles Hurteau and Dr. Dilip Patel, to name two. Finally, I needed and am grateful for the stimulus provided by students and junior physicians who seldom failed to ask embarrassing questions that forced me to think further. The answers are elusive.

Contents

Part Three   Topics Important to Those with Gut Reactions

PART ONE

Understanding the Gut

CHAPTER ONE

The Gut

A Guided Tour

I hav finally kum to the konklusion, that a good reliable set ov bowels iz worth more to a man, than enny quantity ov brains.

Henry Wheeler Shaw [Josh Billings] (1818–1885)

We call it the gut. *Gut* is an old Anglo-Saxon word that applies to the passage from the mouth to the anus. *Intestine,* like many Franco-English words, may appeal to the sensitive, but it excludes the stomach and the esophagus. *Bowel* and *intestine* refer only to the lower gut. The *digestive, alimentary,* or *gastrointestinal tracts* may get around some of the difficulties of the other terms but also include the pancreas and the liver. Seldom are these terms used outside medical meetings. Perhaps the word *gut* is less objectionable nowadays; it is, after all, the title of a distinguished British medical journal.

Because this chapter briefly outlines the anatomy of the gut, many terms appearing here will be used throughout the book. But no attempt is made to describe the parts of the gut in any detail or to state the relationships of the gut to other organs. Like all living tissue, the gut is made up of cells. The study of cellular tissue, which is called *histology*, can only be performed with a microscope. The histology of the gut is very complex, and since histological abnormalities are not found in the gut reactions that will be described in this book, little reference to it appears here.

STRUCTURE OF THE GUT

At autopsy, the human gut is 9 meters (30 feet) from mouth to anus. In the living person, the tone of gut muscle contracts it to about one half of that length. Although the mouth and throat are part of the gut, our description will begin at the esophagus (gullet) and continue through the stomach, the small intestine, the colon, the rectum, and the anus.

The gut is a hollow, very flexible tube, the wall of which has three layers: an outer coating called the *serosa*, a muscular layer called the *muscularis*, and an inner lining called the *mucosa* (Figure 1). The serosa coats the intra-abdominal organs, stomach, small bowel, and colon, which are arranged within the chest and abdominal cavity as shown in Figure 2.

The gut is a dynamic organ almost always on the move, and its driving force is the gut muscle. There are two muscle coats. The outer, thinner layer consists of muscle cells or fibers arranged longitudinally. In the colon, this layer becomes three longitudinal bands called *teniae coli*. The longitudinal layer shortens and lengthens the gut as it moves its contents along. The inner, circular layer becomes thickened or specialized at various points to form one-way valves or *sphincters*. Circular muscle contractions coordinate with longitudinal contractions to cause a ripplelike movement that carries the intestinal contents along the gut—a process known as *peristalsis*. In the colon, the circular muscle may cause segmental contractions that halt the progress of feces or that move it back and forth to encourage mixing and metabolic interaction with colon bacteria and mucosa. Gut muscle from the midesophagus to the anus is referred to as *smooth muscle* and is under involuntary con-

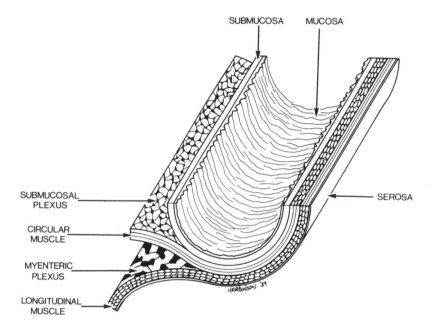

Figure 1. The layers of the intestinal wall. Note that the submucosal nerve plexus (network) lies between the submucosa and the circular muscle. The myenteric plexus lies between the two muscle layers. In the small intestine, semicircular folds shown here increase the mucosal surface, maximizing its contact with the intestinal content.

trol. This feature distinguishes it from the skeletal or *striated muscle* in the limbs that is under voluntary control.

The innermost gut layer, the mucosa, is also dynamic, although in a metabolic sense. The mucosa is a single layer of cells that are specialized to handle water, minerals, and nutrients. Beneath this cellular layer or *epithelium* is the *submucosa*, containing a variety of cells which handle absorbed nutrients, or which play a role in the defense of the body against unwanted invaders, such as viruses, bacteria, or toxins.

The *gastric* (ie, stomach) mucosa produces a fluid so strongly acid that it will burn other tissues. For example, you may expe-

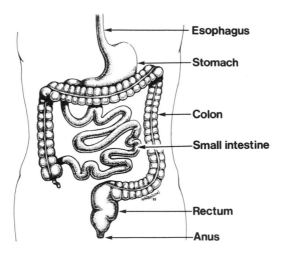

Figure 2. The gut showing the relationships of the stomach, small intestine, and colon within the abdominal cavity.

rience a burning in the throat when you vomit. This same acid (*hydrochloric*) is called *muriatic* acid by bricklayers, who use it to clean mortar from bricks. Thus, the mucosa of the stomach and upper small intestine must be metabolically tough enough to resist destruction by the acid and by a protein-digesting enzyme called *pepsin*, otherwise ulceration occurs.

The small intestinal mucosa is responsible for the absorption of most nutrients and the daily exchange of about 8 liters of fluid entering the gut from ingestion, or from secretion from the intestine, the pancreas, and the liver. The pancreatic and bile ducts empty pancreatic juice and bile from the pancreas and the liver into the upper small intestine. To maximize this enormous fluid exchange, the small intestinal mucosa is pleated into semicircular folds (Figure 1). The epithelial cells are arranged in long fingerlike projections into the lumen called *villi*, which can be seen with the microscope. To even further increase the gut's luminal surface, each cell has tiny projections called *microvilli*, which are seen only through the electron microscope.

SUPPORT SYSTEMS

Because the gut cannot function on its own, it must communicate with the rest of the body for the transport of nutrients, gases, and chemical messengers, and for regulation. Three large arteries, the *celiac*, the *superior*, and the *inferior mesenteric*, arise from the aorta to supply oxygen and other nutrients to the stomach, the small intestine, and the colon (the intra-abdominal gut). Corresponding *veins* carry away absorbed nutrients and gases in a process that is so efficient that hydrogen gas produced by the action of colon bacteria on intestinal contents appears within seconds in the breath. Tiny vessels called *lymphatics* carry absorbed fats from the small intestine to the circulation.

Gut regulation is accomplished by the *enteric nervous system* (ENS) and by an ever increasing list of hormones and *neurotransmitters* that have complex effects on gut movement and fluid transport through the mucosa. The ENS is a complex network of nerves and ganglia within the gut wall. The nerve network that is found between the circular and the longitudinal muscle layers is called the *myenteric plexus;* that between the muscle and submucosa is called the *submucosal plexus*. Through connections to muscle, mucosa, and blood vessels, this "gut brain" governs our digestion. The ENS communicates with the brain, first, via the *sympathetic nerves* that pass to and from the gut through transformers called *sympathetic ganglia* (Figure 3). These nerves connect to the spinal cord and then to the base of the brain. Second, *parasympathetic nerves* connect with the base of the brain via the vagus nerve from the upper gut or the sacral nerves from the colon. Each nerve transmission is affected by one of several neurotransmitters or hormones acting upon an appropriate receptor in muscle or in nerve ganglion. Most of these chemicals are also found in the central nervous system (brain and spinal cord). Later, in Chapter 20, we will note how some drugs act by mimicking neurotransmitters at their receptors. It is said that the complexity of the ENS or gut brain is nearly equal to that of the central nervous system. From this discussion, it is clear that the brain and the gut are intricately interconnected and,

Central Nervous System (i.e. Brain)

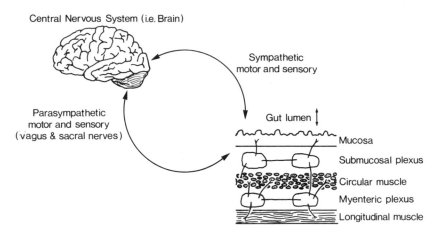

Figure 3. The enteric nervous system (ENS) lies within the gut wall and, through the sympathetic and parasympathetic nerves, transmits and receives information to and from the brain.

for our purposes in this volume, it is well to remember that events in the one are unlikely to be ignored by the other.

Esophagus

The esophagus (or gullet) is 20 to 22 centimeters (8 or 9 inches) long (Figure 4). It begins where the pharynx or throat ends, below and behind the Adam's apple. Here the *cricopharyngeal* muscle, a striated muscle under voluntary control, forms the first gut sphincter, which is called the *upper esophageal sphincter* (UES). This muscular valve must relax before food can be admitted to the gut. A dysfunction here is believed to be responsible for the globus sensation (see Chapter 8). The body of the esophagus is powered by striated muscle in its upper third and smooth muscle in the remainder. More than a passive tube, the esophagus carries food through peristalsis, thus explaining how the opposum hangs in

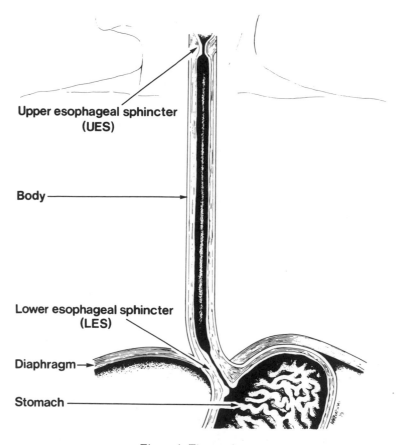

Figure 4. The esophagus.

there without getting up for dinner. At the lower end, there is another valve, the *lower esophageal sphincter* (LES), which must relax as food arrives. Normally, the LES is located at the diaphragm where the gut enters the abdomen. Dysfunctions of the body of the esophagus and lower esophageal sphincter may cause chest pain or heartburn (see Chapters 9 and 10).

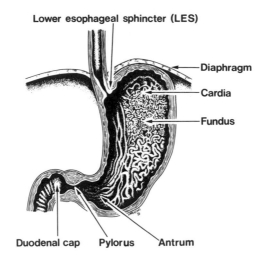

Lower esophageal sphincter (LES)

Diaphragm

Cardia

Fundus

Duodenal cap   Pylorus   Antrum

Figure 5. The stomach.

Stomach

The stomach (Figure 5) is tripe to the butcher, haggis to the Scot, and a favorite scientific frontier for the physician. Its mysteries are still being unraveled. It is curious that an organ about which so much has been written is not essential for life. With altered eating habits, nutritional care, and vitamin B_{12} injections, patients whose stomachs have been surgically removed have been known to live for many years. Nonetheless, the stomach stores and mixes a meal, begins the digestive process, and is the putative source of many digestive complaints including dyspepsia (see Chapter 12).

The stomach is a variably shaped organ, resembling somewhat a fat reclining J, and is comprised of three parts: the *cardia*, which lies above the *fundus,* which extends from the cardia vertically downward, and the *antrum,* which is the foot of the J-shape ending at a thickened muscular ring called the *pylorus.* The upper stomach can be regarded as a container, whereas the antrum has mixing

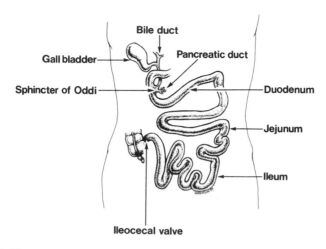

Figure 6. The small intestine. Note that the duodenum becomes the jejunum at the ligament of Treitz and that pancreatic juice, containing digestive enzymes, and bile, containing bile salts, enter the duodenum at the sphincter of Oddi.

and pumping actions. The circular muscle layer of the stomach is separated from that of the duodenum by the pylorus, the third valve or sphincter that is encountered in the gut.

Small Intestine

As mentioned, the small intestine (Figure 6) plays the major role in the absorption of nutrients. It is attached to the posterior wall of the abdomen by the *mesentery*, a ligament that contains the major blood vessels, nerves, and lymphatics. There are three major segments within the small intestine: the *duodenum*, the *jejunum*, and the *ileum*. The first part of the duodenum, which is just beyond the pylorus, is called the *duodenal cap*. It is here that duodenal ulcers occur. The remainder of the duodenum encircles the head of the pancreas and ends at a sharp angulation called the *ligament of Treitz*. The *common bile duct* and the *pancreatic duct* originate in the liver

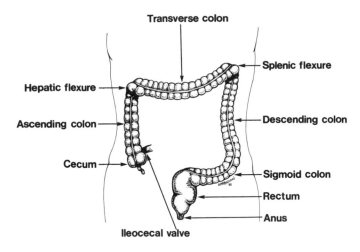

Figure 7. The colon.

and pancreas, respectively, and enter the duodenum at the sphincter of Oddi.

The jejunum is the longest segment of the small intestine and is the most important in terms of the absorption of water, minerals, and nutrients. No feature marks the imperceptible junction of the jejunum with the ileum. The ileum is the site of the absorption of vitamin B_{12} and bile salts, and terminates at the next gut sphincter, the *ileocecal valve*.

The Colon

The Flanders of medicine.

E. I. Spriggs (1930)

Another organ we can apparently do without, the colon (Figure 7) is nonetheless the site of many gut miseries. Much of the pain that is associated with the irritable gut likely originates in the

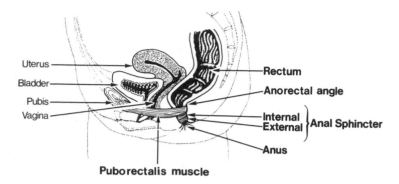

Uterus
Bladder
Pubis
Vagina

Rectum
Anorectal angle
Internal
External }Anal Sphincter
Anus

Puborectalis muscle

Figure 8. The anorectum. The semilunar rectal valves help slow the fecal flow. When rectal distension with stool stimulates the defecation reflex, the puborectalis muscle relaxes, straightening the anorectal angle. The internal anal sphincter relaxes and the descending colon contracts. Defecation is prevented by voluntary contraction of the external anal sphincter.

colon. As depicted in the figure, the colon or large intestine begins at the ileocecal valve with the cecum and the ascending colon. It then travels up the right side of the abdomen, turning at the hepatic flexure, and crosses the upper abdomen as the transverse colon; then, at the splenic flexure, it descends down the left side of the abdomen to the sigmoid colon and rectum. At this point, it is well to be aware that our colons contain a myriad of bacteria with which we have great interdependence, because the digestive process is completed in the cecum and the right side of the colon by these organisms. Also, up to a liter of water is reabsorbed by the colon, and a semisolid fecal mass remains. The *rectum* acts as a storage container.

The Anorectum

The storage and evacuation of feces and the maintenance of continence are complex topics that will be discussed in more detail in Chapter 2. Here, we will merely point out that the rectum is a spacious organ lying in front of the sacrum and (in the woman) behind the vagina and the bladder (Figure 8). Several anatomical features serve to hold back feces in the rectum, including the sharp anorectal angle, which is maintained by the *puborectalis*, a pelvic floor muscle shown in the diagram. There are also a series of semilunar projections into the lower rectum called *rectal valves*. Finally, there is the *anal sphincter*. In fact, there are two anal sphincters. The inner one consists of smooth muscle and is under ENS control. The external anal sphincter consists of striated or voluntary muscle and can be controlled through toilet training.

SUMMARY

The gut is a 9-meter-long muscular organ that commences at the throat and ends at the anus, and that consists of an outer longitudinal layer and an inner circular layer. The coordinated contractions (peristalsis) of these layers move intestinal contents in a manner programmed by the enteric nervous system in the gut wall, which is, in turn, influenced by neurotransmitters, hormones, and connections to the central nervous system. The mucosa, responsible for the absorption of nutrients and the secretion of acid and enzymes, is also under ENS control. The esophagus is an active muscular conduit with upper and lower esophageal sphincters. The upper stomach acts as a meal container into which acid and pepsin are secreted and where digestion begins. The lower stomach, the antrum, is a pump that grinds food and injects measured amounts of gastric contents through the pylorus into the upper intestine. The jejunum and ileum of the small intestine serve to absorb nutrients, and the ileum terminates in the ileocecal valve. The colon is a bacteria-filled organ that changes semifluid small-intestinal contents into feces. The anatomic configuration of the rectum and anus is vital to normal defecation and continence.

CHAPTER TWO

How the Gut Works

Our digestions . . . going sacredly and silently right, that is the foundation of all poetry . . . the most poetical thing in the world is not being sick.

G. K. Chesterton (1908)

Once swallowed, a *mouthful* becomes a *bolus* that is carried to the stomach, where it is mixed and partly digested into *chyme*. Upon entering the upper small bowel, it becomes *intestinal contents*, which are altered by absorption and secretion through the mucosa. Somewhere further down, this traveling contents becomes feces or stool, certainly in the lower colon and beyond. In order that these metamorphoses occur in an orderly fashion, gut smooth muscle must convey the luminal contents in a suitable manner. This process is governed by the enteric nervous system (ENS) and its neurotransmitters, which, in turn, are influenced by hormones and interconnections with the brain. The motility of the gut is influenced by a variety of reflexes that respond to the concentration, osmolarity, size, and nature of the luminal contents and to events occurring elsewhere in the gut. Thus, when in perfect harmony, various segments of the gut accept food and move it along, extracting the water, salts, and nutrients needed by the body. Ulti-

15

mately a soft, formed, easily passed stool is prepared to be evacuated at a time convenient to the individual. Normally, all this activity occurs without its entering the person's consciousness. However, an awareness of gut activity and a sense of gut dysfunction are the subjects of this book.

This chapter will therefore discuss the manner in which the gut works, that is, its physiology. Because most functional complaints are believed to be due to motor disturbances, we shall concentrate on the smooth muscle function of the various gut segments. When it seems relevant, the physiology of the mucosa, that is, absorption and secretion, will also be mentioned.

THE ESOPHAGUS (GULLET)

The upper esophageal sphincter (UES) is the first one-way valve that the food bolus encounters as it begins its journey down the gullet (even though the mouth might be considered by some to be the first, it is not one-way nor is it involuntary). When food is swallowed, the UES must relax to allow food to pass into the esophagus. There is some evidence that this valve helps to prevent food and gastric juice, which escapes from the stomach into the esophagus, from refluxing back into the throat. Its importance here is in relation to the globus sensation (see Chapter 8).

The body of the esophagus is not a simple conduit. Its inner and outer muscular layers coordinate to produce primary peristalsis—a wave of increased intraesophageal pressure preceded by relaxation. Normally, this wave carries a bolus of food before it into the stomach, a process which takes approximately 7 seconds. It is also normal for the UES to remain open during rapid swallowing of liquids, and only the final swallow stimulates peristalsis—a facility that is critical to the beer-drinking contestant. A bottle inverted over a rapidly swallowing pharynx (throat) discharges itself into the relaxed gullet and the contents are swept forward by peristalsis. With age, peristalsis may occur with only 50 percent of swallows, and there may be nonperistaltic (tertiary) contractions. Distension of the esophagus initiates so-called secondary peristalsis, an important mechanism for clearing the esophagus of foreign bodies or of acid reflux from the stomach. At times, abnormal esophageal motility has been associated with some cases of non-cardiac chest pain (see Chapter 9), and impaired clearing of acid from the body of the esophagus may contribute to heartburn (see Chapter 10).

Anatomists have failed to identify any thickening of the muscle layer that could represent the *lower esophageal sphincter* (LES). However, sensors that record intraluminal pressure have detected a high-pressure zone about 3 centimeters long just above the point where the esophagus empties into the stomach (the *gastroesophageal junction* or *GE junction*). In response to the arrival of a peristaltic wave, this one-way valve relaxes to allow the esophageal contents to be discharged into the stomach. Normally, however, LES pressure, as measured by intraluminal sensors, is greater than the intraluminal pressure of the stomach.

Considerable research has centered on the LES site because it is here that the battle is won or lost against the reflux of acidic gastric contents into the esophagus and the consequences of heartburn or esophagitis. Twenty-four-hour recording has shown occasional lapses in normal subjects in whom LES pressure has fallen below gastric pressure, resulting in acid reflux. However, this condition is quickly overcome by the housekeeping action of secondary peristalsis in the esophageal body and the neutralizing effect of swallowed alkaline saliva.

When part of the stomach herniates (protrudes) through the diaphragm up into the chest, a *hiatus hernia* is the result (Figure 14). At one time, it was believed that the anatomic relationship of the LES to the diaphragm was of primary importance. When a hiatus hernia occurred with heartburn or esophagitis, it was once commonplace to surgically repair the hernia, that is, to secure it below the diaphragm where it belongs—an approach that now seems naive. As discussed in Chapter 10, hiatus hernia and heartburn are each very common and must often occur together by coincidence. Two decades ago, experts declared that incompetence of the LES was unrelated to hiatus hernia, and there was little reason to believe that simply moving the LES from the chest back to the diaphragm would restore sphincter competence. Now, there is recognition that these anatomic relationships are of some importance. The sharp angle (angle of Hiss) at which the esophagus enters the stomach may serve as a flutter valve. The normal intraabdominal location of the LES just below the diaphragm may help prevent it from being overwhelmed by any increases in abdominal pressure.

The esophagus, like the remainder of the gut, is under the control of the ENS. The vagus nerve, which supplies most of the gut, enervates largely through the release of acetylcholine through nerve endings in the esophageal muscle, and it excites muscle activity. Such drugs as bethanechol (Urecholine), which can mimic acetylcholine, are sometimes used to stimulate esophageal peristalsis in patients with gastroesophageal reflux (see Chapter 20). These affects are generally opposed by the sympathetic nervous system, which is mediated by noradrenalin or adrenergic drugs that mimic it.

Hormones also influence the LES. Gastrin, which stimulates stomach acid production, increases LES pressure. Cholecystokinin (CCK) and secretin, which normally stimulate the gallbladder and pancreas, lower LES pressure. On a more practical level, alcohol, nicotine, and chocolate all relax the LES and are known clinically to encourage reflux.

We still do not know the answer to the question whether LES is sufficient to explain the control of GE reflux, but we have made some progress since Hippocrates, who believed that swallowed fluid was filtered by the lungs into the pericardial sac, where it cooled the feverish heart. The notion that the primary symptom of GE reflux should be called *heartburn* has a venerable past.

STOMACH

Gastric Motility

As a storage container, the stomach expands to accommodate a meal with little change in intragastric pressure. Such a fine adjustment of the gastric capacity is regulated by tonic contractions and relaxations. *Volume* or *capacity* contractions last about a minute and involve primarily the proximal (upper) stomach. These contractions control gastric emptying of liquids but not of solids.

In the distal (lower) stomach, peristalsis carries gastric contents to or through the pylorus. The mixing and grinding action of the stomach was recognized by nineteenth-century physicians. One hundred and fifty years ago, Alexis St. Martin, a French Canadian voyageur, suffered an accidental gunshot wound which resulted in an opening of the stomach onto the abdominal wall. This circumstance allowed William Beaumont, a U.S. Army surgeon who cared for him, to observe the to-and-fro motion of food in the stomach. Beaumont's journal makes fascinating reading. At the end of the last century, the American physiologist Walter Cannon used newly discovered x-rays to demonstrate gastric peristalsis—a method that is no longer considered safe. Modern methods employ electrical and pressure sensors that are installed in the stomach or radioactive isotopes that can be detected through the abdominal wall. In the latter technique, gamma-emitting materials label the solids and liquids of the meal. A recording device (gamma camera) is then placed over the stomach to monitor the rate of gastric emptying.

Gastric electrical slow waves occur rhythmically at the rate of 3 per minute, beginning about midstomach. A second event is a spike of electrical discharge superimposed upon a slow wave, which may initiate contraction. Whether or not such a discharge and contraction occur in time with the slow wave depends upon the activities of the ENS and the influence of hormones.

Gastric peristaltic waves begin at midstomach and spread as a circumferential band through the antrum to the pylorus. The waves are of two types. The first are smaller weak waves that have a mixing function. Larger, more powerful waves have a propulsive as well as a mixing action. After a meal, conditions are such that each electrical slow wave initiates a peristaltic contraction, which therefore occurs at the rate of 3 per minute. The stomach empties liquids selectively while retaining solids of over 2 millimeters. This capacity depends upon the antrum and pylorus acting in concert.

The pylorus can be seen radiographically and endoscopically to open and close. Antral contractions regularly propel gastric contents toward the pylorus through which small amounts are then squirted into the duodenum. Most contents, including larger particles which are unable to pass the pylorus, are retropelled into the proximal stomach through the nozzle formed by the advancing peristaltic wave. In this fashion, the meal is mixed and ground to particles small enough to be acted upon by the intestine.

In contrast to the postmeal state, the fasting stomach undergoes a three-phase cycle: inactivity, irregular contractions, and a terminal, intense peristaltic phase that sweeps all before it into the duodenum. This cycle may take 1 to 2 hours.

Control of Gastric Emptying

With the development of fiberoptic endoscopes, it is possible to observe gastric activity firsthand (Figure 30). One of the fascinations of fiberoptic gastroscopy is to watch a succession of waves begin modestly in the body of the stomach, sometimes fizzle out, end in a crescendo of terminal antral contraction sometimes, which obliterates the view, and occasionally sweeps majestically through the gaping pylorus into the duodenum.

The electrical and mechanical waves associated with gastric emptying are subject to activity in the vagus nerve (parasympathetic) and the sympathetic nerves that regulate the ENS. The parasympathetic neurotransmitter acetylcholine stimulates gastric contractions, whereas dopamine and the sympathetic neurotransmitter norepinephrine oppose contraction. Many hormones influence the system. Gastrin and motilin appear to stimulate gastric emptying, whereas progesterone, secretin, and cholecystokinin oppose it. Through this complex control system many external factors, including the emotions and physical exercise, influence gastric emptying.

Thus, gastric emptying can be delayed by such widely divergent events as rectal distension, immersion of the hand into ice water, excision of the vagal nerve (vagotomy), fear, anger, the luteal phase of menstruation, and even the time of day. The stomach works faster at 8:00 AM than at 8:00 PM, which will surprise those whose minds and bodies seem to function otherwise.

Distension of the stomach appears to be the principal stimulus to gastric emptying, but certain characteristics of the meal can retard it. Hypothetical receptors in the duodenum are sensitive to fat, hypertonic (concentrated) material, and acid delivered from the stomach. When stimulated, these receptors slow gastric emptying. Liquids and solids made more viscous with pectin or guar gum empty at a slower rate (see Chapter 6). Oils introduced into the ileum can also delay stomach emptying.

Further evidence that the control of gastric emptying is finely tuned is shown by the selective emptying of liquids and solids. Nine tenths of a liquid may disappear in an hour, whereas digestible solids may take four times as long. Solid plastic spheres added to a meal are the last to go, and are emptied by an apparently "disgusted" stomach up to 48 hours later. Control of gastric emptying is destroyed if the vagus nerve is damaged. Thus, gastric retention occurs in patients who have a vagotomy or who have diabetes with nerve damage.

Terminal antral contractions and duodenal contractions must be coordinated to prevent retropulsion of duodenal contents into the stomach. During a meal, the duodenum contracts in time with antral contractions, enabling any gastric content that passes the pylorus to be swept away. Increased concentration of duodenal contents causes increased intraduodenal pressure, which forces the contents away from the stomach. Some reflux of duodenal contents into the stomach normally occurs, and this is exaggerated in persons who smoke and in some patients with dyspepsia. Some experts believe, therefore, that antroduodenal dysfunction may be responsible for upper gastrointestinal symptoms (see Chapter 11).

Thus, the stomach may be regarded as a receptacle, a mixer, and a grinder. The pylorus is the gatekeeper of the intestine, controlling the rate and form in which food is presented for digestion. Its function is subject to many external influences, the composition of its contents, and the activity of the ENS. The ENS, in turn, is subject to central and hormonal control. That a dysfunction of this system *might* cause symptoms, such as dyspepsia and abdominal pain, cannot be denied. As we shall see in Chapters 11, 12, and 13, the nature of this putative dysfunction has not been clearly identified.

SMALL INTESTINE

"Local stimulation of the gut produces excitation above and inhibition below the excited spot." This is the law of the intestine, expounded by the pioneering physiologists W. M. Bayliss and E. H. Starling in 1899. Like most laws, this one is subject to interpretation, and many investigators have since tried to rewrite the legislation.

Because analysis of small-bowel motility is complex, it cannot be dealt with in detail here. Basically, there are nonpropulsive and propulsive contractions. The former, which are discoordinated and occur at adjacent sites in the intestine, move the gut contents back and forth in pendulum fashion. The contractions are most active following a meal, and serve to mix the intestinal contents and ensure maximal contact with the absorbing surface of the mucosa.

In the period between meals, there are cycles of propagating contractions lasting from 2 to 2½ hours. These are the *migrating motor complexes* (MMC), which correspond to small intestinal peristalsis. This peristalsis is characterized by a moving ring formed by circular muscle contraction preceded by relaxation. The role of the MMCs and peristalsis is to keep the small gut clear of residual food and help limit bacterial growth. In addition, there are infrequent powerful or giant migrating contractions that originate in the distal small bowel and sweep through the colon into the rectum. They usually precede defecation and correspond to the "mass movements" described radiographically in the colon (see below). Early in this century, peristaltic rushes of barium were vividly described by Walter Cannon, and are familiar to radiologists. Segmentation and peristalsis are functions of the circular muscle coat, whereas the longitudinal layer is responsible for volume control and the sleeving action of the gut. Reverse peristalsis probably does not occur normally, because electrical impulses are transmitted only toward the rectum.

Large retrograde contractions in the upper small bowel empty the organ into the stomach as a prelude to vomiting. There is, however, no small-bowel correlate to nausea. So far, there is some but little evidence that abnormalities of small intestinal contractions are responsible for symptoms. Emotion or physical stress can alter small-bowel motility, perhaps uniquely so in the irritable bowel syndrome (IBS). Patients with IBS may have their pain reproduced by balloon distension of the small and the large bowel. MMCs may be more frequent and cover a greater length of gut in diarrhea. Powerful migrating ileal contractions that are spontaneous appear to coincide with cramps in the IBS. These snippets of information seem to implicate the small bowel in the irritable gut, but there is much more to learn about the specificity and relevance of these observations.

Not to be forgotten is the remarkable exchange of fluids, minerals, and nutrients across the mucosa. It is estimated that the small intestine handles up to 8 liters of fluid from ingestion and from secretion by stomach, intestine, liver, and pancreas. In cholera, for example, absorption by the small intestine is blocked by the cholera toxin, and the result is severe diarrhea, dehydration, and, if left untreated, will result in death. Small alterations in this extensive fluid exchange could play a role in functional constipation or diarrhea. Generally speaking, laxatives increase net small-bowel secretion, whereas antidiarrheal agents decrease it (see Chapter 19).

COLON

The colon accepts about a liter of liquid from the ileum each day. During passage of this material through the colon, most of the fluid is absorbed, and semisolid feces are presented to the rectum. In steady perfusion studies, up to 7 liters may be absorbed in 24 hours, but much less if the fluid is presented in boluses, such as after meals. Colon bacteria alter the solid portion by the digestion of nonabsorbed glycoproteins and carbohydrates, such as cellulose. Hydrogen, carbon dioxide, and methane gases are produced along with volatile fatty acids, which have both cathartic and nutritive functions. These are absorbed or expelled, and the final fecal mass is mainly water with the major solid component consisting of bacteria (see Chapters 7 and 12).

The movements of the colon may be compared to the Russian empire before *glasnost*—"a puzzle inside a mystery wrapped up in an enigma." There appear to be two basic intermittent myoelectric slow waves: the most prominent has a frequency of 6 to 12 waves per minute. A lesser one of 3 waves per minute may be more frequent in the IBS (see Chapter 13). With the use of a different technology, short and long bursts of electrical activity can be observed. The short bursts appear to be related to mechanical contractions in the colon and may coincide with abdominal pain and constipation in the irritable bowel.

Early in the twentieth century, before the dangers of x-rays were known, a succession of distinguished investigators observed the passage of radiopaque material through the colon. From their work and also the recent use of intracolonic pressure-sensing devices, a concept of colon motility has slowly emerged. There are three modes of colon motor activity. The first mode is basic tone superimposed upon which is the second: the nonpropulsive segmenting contractions. The third mode is the mass propulsive activity that was discussed above in the section dealing with the small intestine. The dominant colon movement is nonpropulsive segmentation, which is most vigorous in the descending colon and sigmoid. These contractions may occur randomly or may be coordinated, but their propulsive activity is minimal.

Radiologically observed mass movements in the colon occur in response to an unknown force. Unlike true peristalsis, a mass movement is apparently not caused by a migrating contraction ring preceded by relaxation. Because they are infrequent, mass movements are difficult to study. After a segment of colon has kneaded the feces for several hours, segmental contractions disappear and the bolus is mysteriously moved on.

Studies of colon motility in humans have been hampered by many methodological limitations. In most instances, pressure and electrical recording devices have been placed only in the sigmoid and the rectum. Different recording devices have therefore produced conflicting results by different observers, and there is controversy as to whether such studies should be conducted in a normal or in an enema-cleaned colon. In patient studies, the symptoms have not been clearly defined, and so we cannot confidently link them to physiological phenomena.

Nevertheless, many researchers suspect that the abdominal pain and altered bowel habit of the IBS are due to colonic dysmotility. Spasm of the colon has been blamed for abdominal pain and constipation since 1830, when John Howship, a British physician, published an article entitled "Spasmodic Stricture of the Colon as an Occasional Cause of Confinement of the Bowels." Since then, several observers have described an almost sphincteric action of the sigmoid colon and have presented data suggesting that colon contractions are increased in constipation and abdominal pain and decreased in diarrhea. Unfortunately, this thesis does not stand up under scrutiny. Also it seems that more than the sigmoid is involved in the genesis of symptoms. Even the fact that abdominal pain of IBS patients may be reproduced by balloon distension of segments of the colon or small intestine does not determine whether the symptoms are due to altered motility or to an altered perception of motility.

The observations that mental and physical stress alter colon contractions, and that a meal especially high in fat may stimulate the colon are strong evidence that the central nervous system, the ENS, and hormones play important roles in colon regulation. The mechanisms that tune colon secretion, absorption, propulsion, retropulsion, and segmentation are intricate indeed. Chesterton was correct: our digestions "going sacredly and silently right" *are* poetic.

DEFECATION

Under normal conditions the rectum is empty. Perhaps because of awareness of a full colon or perhaps in response to eating, the descending colon and sigmoid straighten and undergo an integrated contraction that delivers feces into the rectum. Tonic contraction of the internal anal sphincter maintains continence (Figure 8). Rectal distension reflexly relaxes the internal sphincter and contracts the external sphincter. Continence is then maintained by the external sphincter until a person is ready for voluntary defecation. An upright posture and increased intra-abdominal pressure can also cause the external sphincter to contract. The rectum can accommodate 100 to 200 grams before the defecation reflex is initiated, although the small 100-gram stool typically produced by Western man may not provide an adequate stimulus.

With defecation the puborectalis muscle relaxes and descends, removing the 80- to 100-degree anorectal angle. The external sphincter relaxes, and the descending colon contracts pushing the feces through the now funnel-shaped and patent anus. This action should completely empty the left colon, which appears to function independently of the right. Furthermore, this activity is accompanied to a variable extent by abdominal muscle contraction, diaphragm descent, and forced expiration against a closed glottis (straining).

Much has been made of a person's position at defecation, probably influenced by all sorts of factors that only the upright posture and the social complexities of human nature could contrive. Aside from choosing the place and the time, human beings have selected a variety of positions. The virtues of the squat position employed by natives of Southern Europe and the developing world are said to be superior to the sitting position adopted by much of Western society. Some native Africans regard the indoor lavatory with astonishment. One colonial observed that when persuaded to use the toilet, natives stood on the seat and squatted. Furthermore, they evidently used stones for toilet paper with predictable effects on the plumbing. But habitués of the water closet have found that even the relatively civilized squat in an Italian comfort station can be an athletic feat.

At least 20 percent of normal individuals are aware of regular straining at stool. Could excessive straining damage sphincter nerves and muscle and interfere with the defecation reflex? Certainly, the force with which the sphincter may be closed is impaired by age and childbearing. In general, little is known about performance on the toilet since it is not a spectator sport. Perhaps the science of defecation is in need of the expertise of researchers, complete with bathroom movies to clarify these mysteries.

Fecal continence is a uniquely human attribute, as any visit to the farm reminds us. To be sure, there are primeval reflexes that prevent accidental defecation as a consequence of temporary increases in abdominal pressure. But the voluntary retention of feces throughout the third act of *Aida* is a phenomenon that is unique to civilized man. To this end, there are two factors of vital importance. The first is a conscious control over the voluntary muscles of the external sphincter and pelvic floor. Voluntary closure of the external sphincter and contraction of the puborectalis muscle thus sharpening the anorectal angle make the anal canal an empty, narrow slit (Figure 8). The anal mucosa and the cushionlike hemorrhoidal veins are apposed by the sphincter and act as a seal against increases in intra-abdominal pressure. The second continence factor is the very rich sensory innervation of the anal canal within and above the anal sphincter, which allows the individual to distinguish feces from fluids or flatus. When rectal distension relaxes the internal sphincter, it exposes the sensitive anal mucosa to intestinal content. Thus, one may decide whether to drop one's drink and run, or to close the external sphincter, tighten up the puborectalis, and finish that fascinating conversation. Habitual adoption of the latter course may lead to constipation (see Chapter 16).

There are a number of abnormalities that may be important in the irritable gut. Spasm of the puborectalis muscle may be responsible for the brief but breathtaking pain of proctalgia fugax (see Chapter 17). Failure of this muscle or of the sphincter to relax may contribute to constipation as may weak anorectal contractions or lack of sensation of a full rectum (see Chapter 16). Incontinence may result from decreased perception of watery stool in the rectum, loss of the mucosal plug after hemorrhoidectomy, loss of the anorectal angle, or decreased sphincter pressure (see Chapter 15).

SUMMARY

From the stomach distally, the timing of gut smooth muscle contractions is determined by rhythmic electrical activity. Contractions seem to be influenced by the enteric nervous system and are subject to activity in the central nervous system and to hormones.

In response to a swallow, the upper esophageal sphincter relaxes, allowing passage of the bolus into the esophageal body, down the length of which it is carried by peristalsis. The lower esophageal sphincter relaxes with the arrival of the food bolus, thus allowing the peristaltic wave to sweep all before it into the stomach. Impaired tone of the lower esophageal sphincter or incomplete peristalsis may permit acid, pepsin, and sometimes bile to reflux into the esophagus, causing heartburn and, in some cases, esophagitis.

The body of the stomach adjusts the gastric capacity for food by means of tonic contractions and relaxations. Gastric peristalsis begins in midbody and may sweep through into the duodenum or may terminate in a vigorous contraction against a closed pylorus, which helps to mix and grind the food. Gastric peristalsis is stimulated by distension and is inhibited by fat, acid, and other nutrients through their effect on the duodenal nerve receptors. Fluids empty more promptly than solids. Acting in concert, the antrum and pylorus prevent the reflux of duodenal contents into the stomach. Should this mechanism fail, duodenal-gastric reflux may occur and, in some persons, this might result in dyspepsia.

In the small gut, a series of contractions occur 4 to 5 centimeters apart, dividing intraluminal contents into segments, mixing the contents, and maximizing mucosal exposure. The migrating motor complex (peristalsis) consists of a moving contraction ring that travels only a few centimeters.

Nonpropulsive segmentation is more common in the left colon than in the right and may act to slow the progress of colon contents. Mass movements or peristalsis are rarely recognized. A normal bowel movement is thus a balance of these mechanical forces and the amount of fluid presented to and absorbed from the colon.

Lack of coordination is considered by many researchers to cause abdominal pain, diarrhea, constipation, and other symptoms found in the irritable gut.

Defecation is initiated when contraction of the left colon delivers feces into the rectum. Rectal distension relaxes the internal anal sphincter, but continence can be voluntarily maintained by the external sphincter, which squeezes the anal mucosa and hemorrhoidal venous cushions shut. With defecation, the pelvic floor (puborectalis) relaxes and descends, removing the sharp angle between the anus and the rectum. The descending colon contracts, delivering feces through the funnel-shaped and patent anus. Abnormalities of this complex mechanism are believed important in constipation, diarrhea, and proctalgia fugax.

CHAPTER THREE

Bowel Habit

Human beings have landed on the moon, conquered smallpox, and explored the secrets of the proton, yet they have an astonishing ignorance of their own bowels. With the possible exception of the weather, no subject is so prone to uninformed comment. Before discussing disordered bowel habit, we must first understand what is normal habit. Much of what we know does not result from detailed observation but rather from surveys entirely dependent on the recall of the respondents. As we shall see, consideration of normal and abnormal bowel habit must include not only the frequency of defecation but also the consistency and weight of the stool, and, most importantly, the effort required to defecate. Measurement of the time it takes a bolus of food to transit the gut may also help us understand bowel habit, but it is not a practical means by which we can define constipation or diarrhea.

FREQUENCY OF DEFECATION

We ha' only twa things to keep in meend, and they'll searve us for here and the herea'ter; one is always to have the fear of the Lord before our ees; that'll do for herea'ter; and t'other is to keep your booels open, and that will do for here.

Old Scottish Physician

The traditional "gut feeling" that one bowel movement per day is ideal appears to have been established in human consciousness since antiquity. However, in 1909, the British physiologist Sir Arthur Hurst felt that daily defecation was merely a matter of convenience and claimed that it was not rare to find healthy people whose bowels moved every third day and others in whom a bowel movement three times a day was usual. William Heberdon, a famous nineteenth-century physician, described two "normal patients," one who had monthly bowel movements and the other who had 12 stools per day over 20 years.

Even now, we do not know the normal limits of human stool frequency. In a 1943 study, only 50 percent of 1,100 British post office employees had daily bowel movements. Fully one quarter of these individuals were taking laxatives regularly. It appears that the frequency of defecation was unaffected by age, occupation, exercise, or water supply. Similar conclusions were obtained in a study of 440 British nurses during World War II, of whom 5 percent were taking laxatives.

It seems that only the British have shown much interest in the bowel movement issue. Of 1,455 London factory workers and individuals on the lists of rural general practitioners, 90 percent reported that they had between 3 movements per week and 3 per day, which is close to Hurst's original estimate, and about 70 percent had daily movements. Seven percent of this group considered themselves constipated, but few of these reported infrequent stools, fewer reported hard stools, and many reported neither. Twenty percent of these subjects used laxatives. It is a tribute to the efficacy of pharmaceutical advertising that very few of the laxative users claimed to be constipated. Two studies published in the 1980s confirmed that 96 percent to 97 percent of individuals in Great Britain (Thompson and Heaton, 1980) and the United States (Drossman et al., 1982) have from 3 movements per day to 3 per week. Even now, laxative use is alarmingly common.

Unfortunately, these studies suffer many drawbacks. First, the samples of individuals are not random and must be extrapolated to whole populations with caution. Second, the individuals who furnished the information had to rely on memory, which may have been faulty. Even under relatively controlled conditions, there may be great day-to-day variation in the frequency of bowel action in an individual. The third drawback of these studies is the lack of provision for the variable circumstances in which people live. Many women, for example, notice a change in bowel habit with menstruation; also vigorous physical activity may cause diarrhea, a phenomenon that may dull the competitive edge of the long-distance runner. Heated indoor plumbing may actually encourage more frequent visits than the cold wooden seats of an outhouse. In addition, there may be ethnic or cultural differences. Whites in the United States take more trips to the toilet than blacks. Rural Africans have more frequent and larger stools than their urban brethren. Finally, most of these studies ignore stool weight and consistency, ease of defecation, and the nature of the diet.

STOOL WEIGHT

Most modern gastroenterologists believe that small, hard, dry, "unit" stools are features of constipation. At the other end of the defecatory spectrum, diarrhea is described as the passage of liquid stools exceeding 300 grams per day. By this criterion, all Ugandan villagers have diarrhea, because they produce more than 400 grams of unformed stool daily. The average stool weight in Ottawa, Canada's capital, is 120 grams. (If Parliament were included, the rest of the nation might consider this an underestimate!)

Many factors influence stool weight. Failure of the small intestine to absorb fluid and electrolytes may produce a large stool. For example, cholera toxin impairs salt and water absorption resulting in high-volume, liquid feces. Malabsorption of fat results in bulky, soft stool. Dietary fiber increases stool weight. It would appear that this "bulking" effect of fiber is due mainly to its water-holding capacity, but bacterial proliferation or the production of fiber metabolites could also have laxative effects.

One study demonstrated that with fiber intake held constant, an outgoing personality or a positive self-image may be responsible for an increase in stool weight. (Introverts have always known this about extroverts.) Generally, patients are unable to judge the weight of their stools, so, for history-taking purposes, stool weight is of little value. Occasionally, a physician may collect a patient's stool for 3 days to calculate the daily weight, which helps to decide the magnitude of the complaint. In Western countries, a weight of more than 300 to 500 grams per day suggests an organic process.

STOOL CONSISTENCY

Diaries in which subjects rate their stool as hard, formed, loose, or watery depend upon observations by individuals who may not use the same yardstick. Furthermore, stool that appears rigidly formed in the toilet bowl might collapse like a cow pie if delivered on a flat surface. In an attempt to provide more objective evidence of stool consistency, a *penetrometer* has been devised. The science (or art) of penetrometry consists of the measurement of the distance traveled into the stool of a standard, pointed, inverted cone, dropped from a standard height. To the relief of anyone who might be called upon to employ it, this device has not come into general use.

Generally, hard stools are features of constipation, whereas loose or watery stools occur in diarrhea.

EFFORT

Ease of defecation is another important consideration. Twenty to forty percent of individuals say that they strain at stool. How does one define straining? The force generated, the time required, and even the position assumed during defecation are important. Pressure generated during defecation in order to push hard, lumpy bits of stool through a reluctant pelvic floor may distend hemorrhoidal veins, pop hernias, and cause gastric contents to reflux into the esophagus. The opposite, of course, is lack of straining. In diarrhea, urgent call to stool is often reported. There may be *incontinence* (accidental loss of feces) with soiling, perianal soreness, and great mental distress. Under such circumstances, defecation is effortless but hardly satisfactory.

Ease of defecation and consistency are terms used to define constipation and diarrhea. Straining on more than 75 percent of occasions is said to represent constipation, whereas loose, watery stools on more than 75 percent of occasions constitute diarrhea.

TRANSIT TIME

Transit time is the time required for a meal to pass through the gut. As with most apparently simple biological concepts, transit time has proven to be exceedingly difficult to define and measure. Is the end point to be taken as the appearance of the meal in the stool, as passage of the entire meal, or as passage of some percentage of the meal? Fluids and solids have different rates of transit, so different measuring techniques must be used for each. The emptying time of each segment of the gut may not be in proportion to total transit time. Further, there is evidence that gastric, small-bowel, and colon emptying are controlled somewhat independently.

The earliest record of transit time measurement appears to have been an observation in 1840 of a patient who swallowed a 3-inch piece of a flute, which took 4 days to pass. Serious attempts at measurement began in 1907, with Sir Arthur Hurst, who recorded the transit time of bismuth, which stained the stool black. However, bismuth also causes constipation. Since then, all sorts of substances, from millet seeds to ball bearings, have been employed in various measurement attempts. F. Hoelzel, in 1930, studied transit in a veritable Noah's ark of animals in order to determine that transit time of a substance varies with its specific gravity. Among such items as rubber, cotton, thread, seeds, glass beads, aluminum, steel, silver, and gold, it is the heavier articles that have slower transit.

Transit studies are further complicated by intraluminal mixing. In one experiment, it was found that 75 percent of 50 glass beads passed through in 1 to 4 days, but in one case the last bead appeared on day 40. When beads are given in 2 successive days, those of the second day often appear before those of the first. It is now realized that the high specific gravity of the beads delays their transit. Since the stool must be sieved in order to retrieve the beads, this particular measurement method never caught on anyway.

Dyes, such as carmen red or charcoal, have been used to signal the passage of a test meal. These methods depend upon recognition of the marker in the stool and do not allow for mixing and streaming. The use of chemical markers adds the necessity of quantitative analysis to the difficulties of stool collection.

The use of x-rays to determine transit time is unjustified. However, gamma-emitting isotopes, such as technetium sulfur colloid, have been employed through abdominal scanning to measure gastric emptying. A radioisotope capsule offers an accurate localization while in the gut and a distinct end point when it leaves. Both large and small intestinal transit can be measured by such a device. It is important that the specific gravity of these markers be similar to that of feces, which is about 1.1.

Perhaps the most acceptable and practical measurement of transit time is the hydrogen breath test. Complex carbohydrates, including disaccharides not normally digested in the small gut, are attacked by intestinal bacteria upon arrival at the cecum. The resulting reaction releases hydrogen, which is absorbed and quickly excreted in the breath. Thus, the hydrogen breath test is a reliable indicator of mouth-to-cecum transit. Lactulose, a disaccharide, is the preferred carbohydrate substrate (see Chapters 12 and 19).

The most practical measurement of whole-gut transit time employs plastic radio-opaque pellets. The time required for 80 percent of 20 of these nontoxic bits to be detected by x-ray of the stool is declared the "80 percent transit time." In normal men, transit varies from 50 to 150 hours, a wide range indeed! Nonetheless, the method has proven effective in large epidemiological studies. Burkitt used this method in the landmark study of stool weights and transit times of several African and Western populations (see Chapter 6).

Because of variations that are related to intra-intestinal mixing and individual bowel habit, scientists are seeking more accurate transit measurement. Volunteers in Cambridge, England, consumed five pellets per meal in a controlled diet over a period of 4 to 6 weeks (Cummings *et al.*, 1976). Researchers collected all stools, x-rayed them, and calculated the mean transit time. There were fluctuations in transit during this period, but the mean was 2 to 3 days. This is probably the most reliable figure to date. The addition of 35 grams of bran to the daily diet reduced the mean transit time to 1.6 days.

The reader may well ask how useful such a test might be in practice. Few North American subjects would be sufficiently disciplined to take a standard diet with pellets for 6 weeks, while collecting and packaging every stool. Efforts to simplify the collections have not improved acceptability. Although the concept of transit time is important, its measurement is of little practical importance to individual patients.

Studies of transit in various populations, such as those of Burkitt and his colleagues, may shed some light on the relationship of certain diets or diseases to transit (see Chapter 6). It seems that transit varies inversely with dietary fiber intake. Many researchers feel that the fiber deficiency of Western diets, by reducing stool bulk, encourages development of certain conditions, such as constipation, diverticular disease, and the irritable bowel. Determination of the factors that influence transit may help us understand and treat these conditions. Although of little practical use, the study of gastrointestinal transit, like that of urban transit, is likely to occupy researchers for years to come.

SUMMARY

Normal bowel habit like beauty "often lies in the eye of the beholder." A person may erroneously believe that he has diarrhea if he passes several stony, hard pellets daily, while another believes he is woefully constipated if he spends a day without defecation. Only considerations of frequency, consistency, *and* ease of defecation should be used to decide if a subject has diarrhea or constipation. In doubtful cases, measurement of daily stool weight provides supplementary information.

Transit time is an important concept if we are to understand altered gut function. Methods of transit measurement are too cumbersome for clinical practice, and only continuous stool collection, using pellets as markers, is reliable for whole-gut transit. The lactulose breath test is a simple method of estimating mouth to cecum transit.

For population surveys or clinical trials, the following definitions of constipation and diarrhea may be useful. Diarrhea is the passage of loose, watery stools on more than 75 percent of occasions, correlating also with the presence of urgency and more frequent stools. Constipation is straining at stool on more than 75 percent of occasions. It also occurs with scybalous (hard) stools and less frequent defecation. Even in the space age, we have improved little on the observation of Hippocrates:

> It is best when the stools are soft and formed and passed at an hour customary to the patient when in health.

CHAPTER FOUR

Symptoms and Syndromes

Physicians think they do a lot for a patient when they give his disease a name.

Immanuel Kant (1724–1804)

Thus far, we have discussed the anatomy and physiology of the gut and the concept of normal bowel habit. As we turn our attention to disturbed bowel function, that is, the irritable gut, some definitions are necessary. In this chapter, we shall discuss the definition of the irritable gut and introduce its symptoms and syndromes.

The irritable gut is sometimes called *functional bowel disease*. A working group of the 13th International Congress of Gastroenterology in Rome presented the following definition:

> A variable combination of unexplained, chronic or recurrent gastrointestinal symptoms not explained by structural or biochemical abnormalities. These may include symptoms attributable to the esophagus, stomach, biliary tree, small or large intestines or anus. (Thompson *et al.*, 1989)

Since the gut appears to react to events in the sufferer's environment, the resulting symptoms and syndromes might be considered to be *gut reactions*.

A *symptom* is a sensation experienced only by the individual. It is intensely private, in the sense that the feeling can only be shared verbally. If a person has swollen legs or blue lips, these *signs* may be seen by a doctor or others. A symptom such as pain has no objective measurement and cannot be observed. Suffered in silence or with outward anguish, others know of the pain only by what the sufferer describes. The irritable gut is characterized by symptoms without signs. No amount of examination, blood tests, or x-rays will disclose a finding that all would recognize and that would allow one to declare "Aha, he has an irritable gut." The personal experience of the irritable gut sufferer introduces a fundamental tenet of this book. You may tell your doctor you have shortness of breath, chest pain, and swollen ankles, and upon examination he will accurately determine whether or not you have heart failure. In fact, he may diagnose the heart trouble during a routine examination even if you don't tell him anything. This is not the case with the irritable gut, where silent sufferers may take their life-long symptoms to the grave.

A *syndrome* is a set of concurrent symptoms that may be recognized as a disorder or disease. Within the irritable gut, there are several syndromes that physicians may recognize from a patient's description of his symptoms (Table 1). In fact, the irritable gut may be considered a spectrum of syndromes believed, *but not proven,* to be due to disturbed gut physiology at sites from the gullet to the anus (Figure 9). Thus, globus may be due to a disturbance of upper esophageal sphincter function, and dyspepsia may be due to disordered stomach emptying. Again, it is important that the nosology of the irritable gut depends upon the words of sufferers and not on any measurement by a second party. (By the way, a *nosologist* is not a nose specialist but a person who classifies diseases.)

SYNDROMES

Although each syndrome will be discussed more extensively in later chapters, here the syndromes and their several symptoms

Table 1
Symptoms and Syndromes[a]

Syndromes	Prevalence (% of total)	Symptoms	Prevalence of healthy adults (%)
Globus	45	Lump in the throat	45
Irritable esophagus		Chest pain	
		Difficulty swallowing	
Heartburn	34	Heartburn	34
Nonulcer dyspepsia	7	Postprandial epigastric pain	3
		Belching	
		Bloating/distension	30
Burbulence		Borborygmi	58
		Abdominal pain	
		Farting	
Irritable bowel		Biliary pain	
Chronic abdomen		Abdominal pain relieved by	14
		defecation; altered	7
		frequency, and consistency	8
Constipation	8	Straining	39
		Scybala	39
		Mucus	5
		Feeling of incomplete	50
		evacuation	
Diarrhea	5	Loose/watery stools	33
		Urgency	31
		Incontinence	
Proctalgia fugax	14	Rectal pain	14

[a] Prevalence figures reproduced with permission from *Gastroenterology* (1980;79:283–288) and *Canadian Medical Association Journal* (1982;126:46–48).

are simply introduced and defined. Note that these syndromes overlap each other, and some symptoms occur in several syndromes. Individuals may have more than one syndrome, or, in some cases, exact classification may not be possible.

Globus is a ball or lump in the throat. Often confused with *dysphagia* (difficulty swallowing), the globus sensation occurs between meals and thus allows the sufferer to eat normally. The *irritable esophagus* is chest pain alleged to emanate from the esophagus.

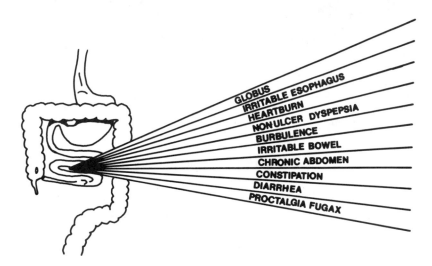

Figure 9. The irritable gut may be considered a spectrum of syndromes and symptoms emanating from gullet to anus.

Noncardiac chest pain in a person is infrequently proven to have an esophageal source, yet the esophagus remains suspect. Should dysphagia occur with the pain, attribution to the esophagus is more convincing. *Heartburn* is a burning retrosternal discomfort or pain often made worse by the consumption of certain foods, emotion, bending, or reclining.

Dyspepsia defys accurate definition. It is often equated with indigestion, a term which is even more imprecise and will not be used further. For our purposes, dyspepsia will be defined as chronic or recurrent, often meal-related, upper abdominal (epigastric) pain, which the physician suspects may be due to a peptic ulcer. *Nonulcer dyspepsia* (NUD) is a functional disorder characterized by dyspepsia in which no ulcer is found. *"Burbulence"* refers to gassy symptoms that may include *belching,* a feeling of *abdominal fullness, bloating* or *distension,* and *farting.* These symptoms are very common in the population and often accompany dyspepsia and the irritable bowel. *Borborygmi* are the bowel sounds that are heard by the individual, and, so he fears, by his friends and colleagues.

This embarrassing noise is so common that it is scarcely abnormal and has no diagnostic importance. It is frequently complained of in several of the irritable gut syndromes.

The irritable bowel is the prototype irritable gut syndrome. It has sometimes been called the *spastic colon* or *irritable colon*, but these terms are now obsolete. At the Rome International Conference (Thompson *et al.*, 1988), it was defined as

> a functional disorder attributed to the intestines:—abdominal pain;— symptoms of disturbed defecation [urgency, straining, feeling of incomplete evacuation, altered stool form (consistency) and altered bowel frequency/timing];—bloatedness/distension.

The chronic abdomen refers to chronic or recurrent abdominal pain not associated with eating or defecation. Many physicians feel that this syndrome is not due to dysfunction of the gut itself but rather a disturbance at the other end of the gut–brain axis (ie, a depression or other emotional disorder). A subset of patients with the chronic abdomen are those whose pain is in the right upper quadrant of the abdomen and which resembles biliary colic. Some persons may have motility abnormalities of the bile ducts that justify the term *biliary dyskinesia*.

As discussed in the previous chapter, *constipation* and *diarrhea* may be defined in terms of frequency, consistency, effort, or transit time. In this book, constipation will be defined as straining at stool on more than three quarters of occasions. Movements may occur less than 3 times a week and may be soft or hard and pelletlike (scybala). *Diarrhea* is loose, watery stools on more than three quarters of occasions. Movements may occur 3 or more times a day and are often accompanied by *urgency*. *Incontinence* is uncontrolled defecation that ranges from fecal soiling of an individual's underwear to complete loss of control. Soiling is often a troublesome but unstated component of diarrhea. The irritable bowel, and sometimes constipation and diarrhea, may be accompanied by stringy, whitish material in the stool called *mucus* and a sensation of *incomplete evacuation*.

According to the Oxford dictionary, *farting* is an old Anglo-Saxon word "not in decent use." Yet its inevitability was certainly recognized long before 1632; "to send forth wind from the anus." What is a chronicler of the irritable gut to do? He could substitute "passage of flatus or gas" if you are an American or "breaking wind" if you are British, but these euphemisms are awkward and do nothing to launder the reality. Like it or not, farting on both sides of the Atlantic is as much a part of the human condition as breathing, so we might as well call a spade a spade (see Chapter 12).

Proctalgia fugax is a sudden severe pain in the anal area that lasts several seconds or minutes and then disappears completely. It may not be a true irritable gut syndrome because the pain seems to originate in the muscles of the pelvic floor.

ORGANIC VERSUS FUNCTIONAL DISORDERS

If functional disorders are gastrointestinal symptoms for which no biochemical or physiologic explanation exists, what shall we call those disorders that have a pathophysiologic explanation? The Oxford dictionary defines the word *organic* as "producing or attended with alteration in the structure of an organ." This is not an entirely satisfactory definition for our purposes because it fails to embrace those conditions that are due to a biochemical abnormality not detected by visual or microscopic examination of the organ. Lactase deficiency, for example, is a condition in which the enzyme lactase normally residing in the intestinal mucosa is missing (Figure 19). This condition results in diarrhea if the individual drinks milk containing the milk sugar lactose. The deficiency is not a functional disease because the mechanism is well explained, and it is not strictly speaking an organic disease because no structural abnormality can be detected. Despite this disadvantage, the term organic will have to do. It is accepted usage for nonfunctional, somatic (of the body) disorders, and despite the Oxford definition, includes those complaints that are due to biochemical defects, such as lactase deficiency.

Organic and functional may thus be considered opposites with the following caveat: the border between them is shifting. Once an organic explanation is found for a functional disorder, by definition the disorder is no longer functional. Persons who had lactose intolerance prior to its description in 1965 would have been diagnosed as having an irritable bowel. One might think then that the numbers of individuals with functional disorders would shrink as more organic causes are found. The uneasy functional–organic dichotomy provides the first glimpse of one of the enigmas of the irritable gut. Will all functional disorders eventually be found to have organic explanation, or are they, like emotions or tears, simply variations in the human experience?

SUMMARY

As no two persons are exactly alike in health so neither are any two in disease; and no diagnosis is complete or exact which does not include an estimate of the personal character or the constitution of the patient.

                                                Sir James Paget (1885)

The irritable gut may be considered a spectrum of syndromes consisting of symptoms emanating from the gut at various points from the gullet to the anus. These symptoms are private experiences known to the world only by the descriptions of their sufferers. They share an absence of satisfactory physiologic explanation and, to that extent, are enigmatic. As we shall see in the next chapter, these syndromes and their symptoms are very common in our population; so common as to blur the border between normal and abnormal. In many cases, it appears that an individual's reaction to the symptom may be as important as the symptom itself. The phlegmatic may consider it part of life, whereas the anxious or obsessive may regard its explanation as a lifetime quest. Thus, it is said that "what kind of a person has the disease is as essential to know as what kind of disease the person has." Paget quotes an old French saying: "'French physicians treat the disease,

English the patient' so far as this is true it is to the honour of the English." Nonetheless, a precise diagnosis of the irritable gut is important if costly, futile investigation and noxious treatments are to be avoided. Then, the business of dealing with one's unruly gut reactions may commence.

CHAPTER FIVE

The Irritable Gut
Prevalence and Cost

Epidemics have often been more influential than statesmen and soldiers in shaping the course of political history, and diseases may color
the moods of civilizations.

René Jules Jean Dubos

There is a tendency to deprecate functional complaints. Physicians
are trained to get to the organic core of a problem and to understand
disease in terms of its pathology. When there is no structural or
biochemical abnormality, symptoms are difficult to understand. It
is easiest to ignore or dismiss that which is not understood. Thus
the aim in diagnosis is to identify or exclude pathology. The irritable gut is what is left when no organic explanation for gut symptoms can be found. This negative approach to the diagnosis of
functional disease leads to tests and therapy that may be inappropriate and often trivialize patients' complaints (Figure 10). After
all, no one has ever died from an irritable gut.

This chapter presents evidence that in Western countries the
prevalence of functional gut complaints is extensive. Loss of work,
unhappiness, and inappropriate investigation or treatment are far

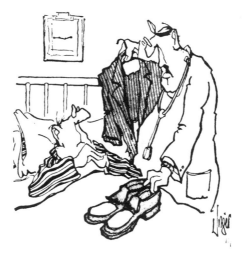

"The results of your tests were negative. Get lost!"

Figure 10. The trivialization of functional complaints. (Herman copyright 1978 Universal Press Syndicate. Reprinted with permission. All rights reserved.)

more common than one might think. In these terms, the irritable gut is not a trivial matter. Upon reviewing such evidence, one can only conclude that the syndromes of the irritable gut are very common entities in their own right and that they deserve positive diagnosis and serious consideration.

PREVALENCE OF THE IRRITABLE BOWEL

Dr. K. W. Heaton and I shared a belief that the irritable bowel is common and that many subjects with such complaints do not report them to their doctors. In order to prove this hypothesis, we administered a questionnaire to 301 healthy British adults (96 percent of those approached). There were roughly 100 in each group of young, middle-aged, and elderly subjects. Twenty-one percent had experienced nonmenstrual abdominal pain at least 6 times in

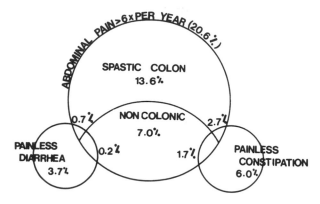

Figure 11. Functional bowel disorders in 91 (30.2 percent) of 301 apparently healthy individuals (nonpatients) with 20 percent having abdominal pain. In 13 percent, the pain was relieved by defecation, and other features of the spastic colon type of irritable bowel were present. In the 7 percent whose pain was unaffected by defecation, the discomfort occurred in the upper abdomen and was meal related. These subjects were said to have dyspepsia. The 6 percent with constipation had straining of stool in more than 75 percent of occasions, whereas the 4 percent with diarrhea had loose, watery stools in more than 75 percent of occasions. Reproduced with permission from *Gastroenterology* (1980:79;283–288).

the previous year, and 13.6 percent had their pain relieved by defecation (Figure 11). This last group usually reported pain in the lower abdomen and were more likely than the remaining subjects to have had several symptoms previously shown to be associated with the irritable bowel (see Chapter 13). When defined as "frequent loose stools," or "frequent straining," diarrhea and constipation occurred in 4 percent and 6 percent of these apparently healthy people. Thus, functional bowel symptoms occurred in 30 percent of the 301 subjects interviewed. Although these subjects were not a true random sample of the population, they were drawn in consecutive fashion from 5 groups of subjects who were not patients. Not only did these results astonish us, they also changed our perspective. Can symptoms that are so common be considered abnormal? Are they, like aging and the menopause, normal facets of the human condition?

The above symptoms are indeed common in Western cultures (Table 2). In North Carolina, Drossman and his colleagues (1982), using a modification of our questionnaire on 789 college students and hospital employees, obtained similar results. Whitehead (1982) interviewed 832 people randomly selected from the Cincinnati telephone directory and identified irritable bowel syndrome (IBS) in 8 percent. Twenty-nine percent of 1,345 Michigan subjects had IBS. Employing our criteria for IBS, studies that were done in France and New Zealand reported that 14 percent of people suffer with the syndrome. Among 202 citizens of Sydney, Australia, 32 percent had variable bowel habits, 8 percent had abdominal pain for 2 weeks or more in a 6-month period, and 5 percent each had constipation and diarrhea. According to these surveys, less than one half of the respondents reported their symptoms to a doctor. Those that did, however, constituted a large part of physicians' practices. Reports from gastroenterology clinics in North America and in Western Europe indicate that 20 percent to 50 percent of referred patients had functional complaints, mainly the IBS (Table 3).

Functional abdominal symptoms are not confined to adults. In one survey, 11 percent of 1,000 British school children suffered abdominal pain 3 times in 3 months that was sufficiently severe as to interfere with their activities. There is some indication that such children are likely to have IBS when they become adults.

In contrast to these observations in Western countries, the syndrome is said not to occur in Uganda. It is also rare among black South Africans living in rural areas; but the prevalence of the syndrome among those blacks living in urban centers is similar to that in Western populations. IBS also appears to be prevalent in the Indian subcontinent and in South America. One Japanese study determined that 7.1 percent of 356 university students and 6.1 percent of 400 company employees had IBS symptoms; another study found them in 20 percent of 2,100 high school students. However, in contrast, these symptoms seem to be rare in China. What is it about Western or "developed" cultures that makes bowels irritable? T. L. Cleave, a Royal Navy surgeon, blamed it on our refined carbohydrate diet, and he treated sailors under his care with bran. Dennis Burkitt demonstrated that Ugandans who eat their native

Table 2

Prevalence of Spastic Colon Type of Irritable Bowel Syndrome (IBS) in Apparently Healthy Individuals

Author	Year	Country	IBS (spastic colon type) (percent)	Percentage of IBS reported to MD	Percentage who are female
Thompson and Heaton	1980	United Kingdom	14	20	59
Drossman	1982	United States	17	46	66
Drossman	1984	United States	10	30	60
Whitehead	1982	United States	8	Males 36	
				Females 49	
Greenbaum	1984	United States	24	48	63
Welch	1985	New Zealand	14	—	50
Bomelaer	1986	France	19	—	53

Note: the "Percentage who are female" values 63 appear aligned with Whitehead (63) and Greenbaum (63).

Table 3
Referrals to Gastroenterology Clinics That Are Functional

Author	Country	Year	Percentage of referrals that are functional
Switz	United States	1976	23
Ferguson	Scotland	1977	31
Fielding	Ireland	1977	52
Manning	England	1977	29
Sullivan	Canada	1983	17
Harvey	England	1983	48
Kruis	West Germany	1984	23

unrefined, high-fiber diet have larger stools and shorter gut transit times than Westerners. Still others might contend that the stresses of modern urban society are at fault.

The social implications of IBS are even more interesting when we consider who among the many sufferers complains to the doctors. The population studies mentioned above suggest that 50 percent to 65 percent of IBS sufferers are women (Table 2). In clinics, the dominance of women with IBS seems to be much greater (Table 4). In contrast, Indians and Sri Lankans who attend physicians for the relief of IBS are only 20 to 30 percent female. Why then are Western women with IBS more likely to become patients than men? Why do Indian women sufferers seem less inclined to see a doctor?

Fifty or more years ago, IBS (or membranous colitis as it was then called) was more common among the upper classes. A study from India indicated that the syndrome was more prevalent in private than in public practice. But in most modern Western states, where some form of health insurance is now in place, it is difficult to determine the importance of social class in IBS prevalence and reporting.

IBS appears to be equally common in young, middle-aged, and elderly healthy Western people, with the exception that constipation is more likely in the old. The mean age of onset is about 29 years (with a range of 1–63 years), and the interval between onset and reporting averages 4 years. Why do the sufferers wait? Do

Table 4
Sex Differences in IBS Patients

Author	Year	Country (city)	Percentage of females	Female to male ratio
Powel	1818	England	100	1
White	1905	England	85	6:1
Hurst	1931	England	80	4:1
Chaudhary and Truelove	1962	England	65	2:1
Fielding	1977	England	66	2:1
Ritchie and Truelove	1980	England	74	3:1
Doteval	1983	Sweden	70	2.5:1
Cann	1983	England	80	4:1
Sullivan	1983	Canada	74	3:1
Thompson	1984	Canada	79	4:1
Mathur	1966	India (New Delhi)	28	1:3
Pimbarkar	1970	India (Bombay)	26	1:3
Bordie	1972	India (Raipur)	18	1:4
Mendis	1982	Sri Lanka (Colombo)	30	1:2

many sufferers report only when reminded of their mortality by a crisis, such as a death in the family?

The large number of people with IBS symptoms who do not report them to doctors may possibly have less severe symptoms. I suspect, however, that severity is a relatively unimportant determinant of health-care-seeking behavior. The recent surveys by Drossman and by Whitehead point out that IBS patients have more features of emotional disturbance or personality disorder than other patients, whereas IBS sufferers who do not see doctors are emotionally similar to controls (see Chapter 7). The above observations force us to consider the roles of culture, sexual inequality, idleness, wealth, fear of serious disease, emotion, and other factors in the patient's decision to seek help.

PREVALENCE OF OTHER FUNCTIONAL
GUT DISORDERS

We found upon interview that 46 percent of young and middle-aged apparently healthy people experience the globus sensation—that is, a lump in the throat unassociated with swallowing (see Chapter 8). This figure in itself should discourage one from using the obsolete term *globus hystericus*. We also noted that of 301 apparently healthy people, one third of men and women experience heartburn at least once a year (see Chapter 10). Ten percent said heartburn occurred weekly, and 4 percent daily. The figures argue against extensive investigation for these benign complaints in the absence of dysphagia, weight loss, anemia, or other symptoms of organic disease.

Upper abdominal pain unrelated to gallstones or defecation is termed dyspepsia and occurs in 5 percent to 10 percent of apparently healthy subjects. In a 1960 British study of 13,000 autopsies, peptic ulcer was found in 14 percent of men and 8 percent of women. About one third of all patients presenting with dyspepsia have no ulcer on endoscopic examination (see Chapter 11). A reasonable estimate of nonulcer dyspepsia prevalence would seem to be about 3 percent to 5 percent.

Proctalgia fugax occurred in 14 percent of 301 noncomplaining British adults (see Chapter 17), and is more common in young women. Like other functional gut sufferers, most do not report the symptom to a doctor. Among 148 Canadian patients with the irritable bowel, peptic ulcer, or inflammatory bowel disease (IBD), the prevalence was 51 percent in women and 12 percent in men. Although the healthy population study suggested a relationship to IBS, proctalgia fugax was found equally in patients with peptic ulcer, inflammatory bowel disease, and IBS. One might conclude that proctalgia fugax is very common, and that those sufferers who have other gut complaints are more likely to report it.

COST AND CONSEQUENCES

In the previous section, we established that irritable gut symptoms are very common among ordinary individuals. In subsequent chapters, we shall see that such symptoms tend to trouble patients for long periods in their lives (Tables 12 and 19). Although they are chronic, functional symptoms, they neither cause any physical harm themselves nor presage a more serious illness. Nevertheless, many sufferers seek medical attention and become patients. Such health care seeking may trigger tests and treatments that are costly and may be more harmful to the patient's well-being than the disorder itself.

In the United States, functional gut complaints account for more physician visits than inflammatory bowel disease (ulcerative colitis and Crohn's disease), and the days in hospital are similar. The use of drugs in this benign, nonlife-threatening, noncrippling disorder staggers the imagination. Six percent of Britons use laxatives at least weekly. In the United States, there are more than 120 over-the-counter medications for constipation for which $368 million was spent in 1982. H_2 receptor antagonists and other equally expensive anti-ulcer medications have been advocated for dyspepsia, whether or not an ulcer is present. The cost of these medications as well as of anticholinergics, tranquilizers, antidepressants, and countless other drugs used for functional disorders must be enormous; yet in few (if any) instances is efficacy proven.

Because of the fear of organic disease, and also the absence of a test that identifies the irritable gut, those sufferers of functional disorders who see doctors undergo much investigation. Of 527 outpatients in a general practice, 24 percent had altered bowel habit, abdominal pain, or rectal bleeding. Although these symptoms are sometimes early presenting features of serious colonic disease, only one polyp (benign tumor) was found in this group. In the remaining 76 percent who were without symptoms, two cases of cancer and three polyps were found. The authors of this report concluded that a self-completed questionnaire that seeks information about symptoms is "of little value in the early detection of colorectal carcinoma." Dent found the above symptoms so frequently among a random sample of people in Sydney, Australia that he came to the same conclusion. In another study of 97 Ottawa outpatients who were referred for barium enema and in whom IBS symptoms were very common, only 18 had organic disease including 11 polyps but no cancer. The complaints of IBS patients (ie, abdominal pain, altered bowel habit, and gas, which are sometimes accompanied by bright red blood from hemorrhoids or fissures) may cause physicians to order investigations to exclude serious abdominal disease. But the yield seems no greater than if asymptomatic persons were similarly tested.

Consultation, upper and lower gut barium x-ray examinations, upper and lower endoscopy, ultrasonography, CT scans, and kidney x-rays are frequently and fruitlessly performed for functional symptoms. Twenty-one of 22 patients with recurrent upper abdominal pain had their pain reproduced by balloon insufflation in the upper gut. This group had 76 consultations, 72 procedures directed at the bile ducts, 53 barium x-ray studies, 25 endoscopies, and 36 abdominal operations, all of which were negative. The average per-patient cost for these procedures was $1,528 in equivalent 1986 Canadian funds. Such a broadside of investigations is not only costly but also dangerous. To be sure, doctors must be cautious of a missed colon cancer in the over-40 patient, but they should also exercise some judgment.

An even more sinister consequence of the irritable gut is unnecessary surgery. Of 119 patients undergoing appendectomy, only 60 had an organ that was inflamed. The patients with normal appendixes were far more likely than those with inflamed appendixes to be female, to have had a severe emotional experience in the 6 months prior to the surgery, and to have continued to have bowel symptoms a year later. For 60 years, authors have lamented that patients with IBS complaints are prone to surgery. In one study, IBS patients underwent 4 times more appendectomies and 3 times more hysterectomies than a similar group with ulcerative colitis. A study in Ireland found that 50 IBS patients, compared to age- and sex-matched controls, were very much more at risk for surgery, repeated surgery, and abdominal surgery. Inquiry often reveals that the operation resulted in the removal of a normal appendix, uterus, or gall bladder and, in the case of multiple surgery, lysis of adhesions. Perhaps it should not be surprising then that 16 percent of IBS patients in one clinic turned in desperation to practitioners of alternative medicine.

CONCLUSIONS

While pondering the prevalence of functional gut symptoms, one editorialist asked, "When exactly do deviations from average bowel function become functional bowel disorder?" When, indeed, does reduced glucose tolerance become diabetes? Almy asked if the IBS is "a qualitative, or merely quantitative departure from the psychophysiological reactions of normal people." That is, is it a disease for which a cause or causes will someday be known, or is it, like tears, a means by which we respond to the environment? It is apparent that severity of symptoms is not the only motive a patient may have for consulting a doctor. Discovery of the cultural, fearful, and emotional factors underlying the visit may provide vital clues as to how the patient may best be helped.

Whatever the cause of the complaints, care of such patients is costly. Clinical and basic research into the nerve–gut interactions of those with and without symptoms may lead to the identification of pathophysiological markers. This would allow inexpensive and reliable diagnosis of functional gut syndromes, reduce morbidity, and save resources for the detection and cure of more serious disease. Although the symptoms of the irritable bowel are not those of cancer or IBD, these diseases may occur coincidentally. Thus, there will always be a need to be alert for the signs and symptoms of organic conditions. Nonetheless, the common functional gut complaints demand a positive, confident diagnosis if the physician is to be believed by the patient, and if costly, unnecessary, and harmful tests are to be avoided.

CHAPTER SIX

The Fiber Story

What thought so wild, what airy dream so light,
That will not prompt a theorist to write?

George Crabbe

HISTORY

The search for a comprehensive explanation for the ills of humanity has led seekers of health down many garden paths. The snake oil peddlers of the nineteenth century touted remedies for everything from constipation to cancer, and faith healers, spiritual and pharmaceutical, continue to profit from the gullible. The credibility of important medical discoveries has been endangered by a tendency to generalize. Thus, with the discovery of cyanocobalamin, vitamin B_{12} injections became a nostrum for complaints ranging from tired blood to bad nerves. Following Sir McFarlane Burnett's exposition of the clonal selection theory, all sorts of conditions were attributed, without evidence, to autoimmunity. The concept of total environmental allergy is an absurd example of this tendency.

The fiber hypothesis, as the implied pathogenetic effect of a low-fiber diet has come to be known, is still just that: a hypothesis. Amid public and professional enthusiasm for the reintroduction of

59

fiber into the diet, Dennis Burkitt has stimulated a great deal of thought and research. It is probable that not all of his conclusions will be borne out by science. Nonetheless, his theory is persuasive, and it is useful to look at its origins, for it is implicated in the irritable gut.

The laxative effect of bran has been known since antiquity. In 430 BC, Hippocrates stated that "wholemeal bread clears out the gut and passes through as excrement, white bread is more nutritious; it makes less feces." This was an astute observation for so long ago. In ancient Rome, white bread was a luxury. The venerable physician Galen rated the nutritional value of bread inversely to its bran content. In the Middle Ages, the filling, indigestible, and laxative nature of wheat bran was known, moving one commentator to say that "browne bread . . . having moch branne . . . fylleth the belly with excrements and shortly desendeth from the stomache" (McCance and Widdowson). For Shakespeare, bran was a derisive epithet: "asses, fools, dolts! chaff and bran" (*Troilus and Cressida* 2.1).

With the advent of the study of nutrition came the knowledge that some proteins, vitamins, and minerals were contained in bran, that is, the cell wall of the wheat berry. During both world wars, the British government, in an attempt to minimize waste, legislated the "national loaf," which contained a high proportion of bran. At the end of each war, there was controversy over the nutritional value of white versus brown bread, but in the House of Lords the conclusion was reached that the country was much less constipated.

Despite the arguments of nutritionists, physicians of a previous generation were convinced that a low-residue diet, free of fiber, was necessary to rest an unstable colon, allowing its tired, irritated muscle to relax. They claimed that the human intestine is short and not designed for a diet containing a large amount of residue. Excess colon content was held responsible for autointoxication, which was believed to be the source of symptoms ranging from headache to insomnia (see Chapter 16). Thus a fiber-free diet was recommended for the ills of many individuals with as much reason as the prescription of bloodletting in an earlier age.

In 1923, one observer thought the desirable effects of a low-residue diet were a long transit time and a desiccated stool, broken into units. Such intentionally induced scybala were believed to be beneficial, a notion diametrically opposed to that of today's "fiberphiles." Thus, it appears that fashion changes in diet and stools as well as in clothes. The miniskirt might last a decade, but medical fads are with us for a generation.

In 1921, A. Schmidt and C. van Noorden in Germany and Kellogg in the United States advocated "indigestible residue" as a prevention and cure for various disorders. In the 1930s, scientists established the laxative effects of natural fiber. This work seems to have been largely ignored; indeed, it was opposed by distinguished prewar gastroenterologists, such as Walter Alvarez. Its possible importance in the etiology of other colon diseases was not even considered. As a result of the writings of Dennis Burkitt and of T. L. Cleave, however, the earlier findings and opinions have been rediscovered.

THE FIBER HYPOTHESIS

The thesis that has greatly altered diet fashion was first outlined in *The Saccharine Disease* by T. L. Cleave. He noted that, during the nineteenth century, more fiber or bran was removed from flour, and the annual sugar consumption increased from 15 to 120 pounds per person. As a result, Cleave contended, our diets are deficient in fiber and laden with refined carbohydrate. The overconsumption of refined foods, he believed, is responsible for many diseases in Western peoples.

As we have seen, brown bread was considered inferior in ancient times, and the craze for whiter and whiter bread has continued to the present. Great effort was expended to whiten the loaf, even to the point of its adulteration with white lead—a practice that evidently died along with the consumers. Some say the introduction of roller-milling of grains around 1880 led to greater separation of bran and still whiter bread. What was not popularly appreciated was that protein, fat, minerals, and vitamins remained

Table 5
Effect of Dietary Fiber on Stools and Transit Times[a]

Population studies[b]	N	Diet	Mean transit time (hours)	Daily stool weight (grams)
United Kingdom naval ratings	15	Refined	83	104
White South African students	100	Refined	48	173
Urban South African school children	500	Mixed	45	165
United Kingdom vegetarians	24	Mixed	42	225
Rural African school children	500	Unrefined	34	275
Ugandan villagers	15	Unrefined	36	470

[a] Adapted from *Lancet* (1972;2:1408–1411).
[b] United Kingdom naval ratings and white South African students on a "refined" (low-fiber) Western diet have relatively long transit times and low stool weight. As the diet contains more fiber, the stool weight increases and the transit time decreases. Africans on an unrefined or high-fiber diet generate much larger stools and have much shorter transit.

with the bran fraction. Finely milled grain had a creamy color caused by carotene (the Vitamin A precursor), which assiduous millers bleached out in deference to the popular taste.

Burkitt and his colleagues, in the best tradition of Livingstone and Stanley, documented stool weight and transit times in Western and African societies (Table 5). They found that Ugandan villagers, ingesting wholly unrefined food, produce 470 grams of stools per day. On the other hand, British naval personnel, consuming a diet claimed by the authors to represent typical British cuisine, produce an average of 104 grams daily. Even African children produce stools 3 times as large as those of sailors in the Royal Navy. The Ugandans have a gastrointestinal transit time of 36 hours as opposed to 83 hours for the fiber-deficient British tars. Canadians and Americans did not participate in these gastrointestinal Olympics, but data from our unit suggest that the average Ottawa stool weight is 130 grams per day.

Diverticular disease, which occurs in 50 percent of septuagenarians in North America and Western Europe, became common at the end of the nineteenth century. The disease is rare in native Africans but common in those descendants of Africans who reside in the United States. We are assured that the irritable bowel is also rare among Africans, but there is little scientific evidence bearing on this matter. It seems common enough among affluent Nigerians.

Investigations have confirmed the relationship of dietary bulk to gastrointestinal transit time and colon intraluminal pressure. Therefore, a low-bulk diet favors slow transit and high intraluminal pressures; such motility changes are said to precede diverticula formation. This is convincing enough to render obsolete the use of a low-residue diet in the treatment of asymptomatic diverticular disease (see Chapter 18). Contrary to the predominant earlier view, Cleave believed that the unnatural low-bulk diet was introduced too recently in evolution to allow the colon to adapt. The result is a variety of motility disorders leading to constipation, irritable bowel, and diverticular disease. The irritable gut may be a price of civilization.

The fiber concept is less convincing when it attempts to encompass many other diseases of civilization. The loaded colon that obstructs the pelvic veins is blamed for varicose veins and hemorrhoids. This situation is aggravated by the straining necessary to pass small, inspissated, fiber-deficient stools (scybala). Five ounces of refined sugar are consumed almost unnoticed by English people each day, yet twenty apples must be eaten to achieve the same caloric intake. Cleave became convinced, therefore, that a refined diet causes dental caries, diabetes, and obesity. Gallstones also have been blamed on alterations in bile-salt metabolism wrought by fiber depletion.

The thread becomes even more tenuous as peptic ulcer, hypertension, gout, hiatus hernia, and acne rosacea are incorporated in the *Saccharine Disease*. Coronary artery disease, says Cleave, is the result of "sugar glut." However, most observers would insist that the origin of each of these disorders is multifactorial. A refined diet is just another factor worthy of investigation.

The average British daily diet contains an estimated 12 grams of dietary fiber, whereas its African counterpart contains 60 grams. This fivefold discrepancy could be narrowed if whole wheat flour, with 9.5 grams of dietary fiber per 100 grams, were substituted for white flour, which contains only one third that amount. In 1977, only 1 percent of bread produced in the United Kingdom was whole wheat, indicating that fiber had not yet captured the hearts of the nation. But since that time, there has been some increase. The average Briton consumes 18 percent of his calories in the form of fiber-free sugar, and 20 percent from white bread from which most of the fiber has been removed.

There are other factors to consider when comparing the environment of rural Africans to that of urban Westerners. Fiber is not a single substance. None of the fiber consumed by Africans derives from wheat. The fiber from African fruits and vegetables is chemically very different from that found in bran. It does not necessarily follow, therefore, that by encouraging whole wheat bread in the West, we are mimicking the African environment.

The evidence that dietary fiber consumption has declined in the past 100 years has not convinced everyone. The figures are based on crude fiber estimates, which we shall see are not credible today. It does appear from the scanty eighteenth-century information available that cereal fiber consumption has fallen, but this is countered by a rise in fiber intake from fruit and vegetable sources. All such information is based on government production figures and cannot include consumption of private garden produce. In truth, we do not know the daily dietary fiber ingestion of 100 years ago. Further, it seems that the average stool weight from 1840 to 1906 ranged from 93 to 150 grams, indicating that while fashions have changed since the Victorian era, stool weights have not.

Nonetheless, some fiber researchers are firmly committed to the thesis that fiber deficiency is harmful to health, and that human beings cannot live by nutrients alone. A British pharmacologist called the introduction of white bread and refined carbohydrate a "major dietary disaster." The place of bran in the treatment of constipation seems secure. It makes sense in uncomplicated diverticular disease, and is probably therapeutic in some cases of the irritable bowel. The role of fiber in health awaits both an accurate definition of its many constituents and well-controlled, long-term studies of their effect on gut function, the incidence of disease, and the metabolism of lipids and other nutrients.

WHAT IS FIBER?

A precise definition of dietary fiber is elusive. Nineteenth-century animal nutritionists considered it a useless constituent of feed. The first scientific attempt to measure "nonnutrients" was an 1806 German method in which the feed was ashed following treatment with petroleum ether, acid, and alkali. The weight of the residue before ashing minus the weight of the ash was termed *crude fiber*. This method is still used to give farmers an indication of the nutritional content of feed, but it is unsatisfactory as a measure of dietary fiber. It detects only lignin and cellulose.

The term *residue* refers to what is left of a meal after digestion, but it ignores bacteria, shed mucosal cells, and secretions. *Roughage*, which refers to material contained in nuts, bran, fresh fruit, and vegetables, is believed to be poorly digested and irritant. *Bulking agents* are those substances that increase stool bulk. Even these terms do not help us understand what is meant by dietary fiber.

In 1929, the term *unavailable carbohydrate* was introduced and was defined as that portion of dietary carbohydrate, including cellulose and hemicellulose, that was not digested by human intestinal enzymes. However, lignin is not a carbohydrate. More recent methods of analysis claim to measure total *dietary fiber;* that is, unavailable carbohydrate plus lignin. Bran is 40 percent dietary fiber by this estimation, but only 10 percent crude fiber. The current working definition of dietary fiber is "endogenous components of plant materials in the diet which are resistant to digestion by human (intestinal) enzymes." It consists mainly of nonstarch polysaccharides and lignin.

Table 6
Components of Dietary Fiber

1. Structural (insoluble)
   Cellulose
   Lignin
   Hemicellulose
2. Nonstructural (soluble)
   Pectin
   Plant gums (guar, karaya)
   Mucilages (psyllium, isbaghula)
   Algal polysaccharides (agar)
3. Other
   Phytate
   Minerals
   Cuticular substances

COMPONENTS OF FIBER

The term *dietary fiber* is misleading because all substances that are encompassed by it are not fibrous. The structural or fibrous components of dietary fiber include cellulose, hemicellulose, and lignin (Table 6). Pectin, gums and mucilages, and algal polysaccharides are nonstructural, more soluble substances. These diverse polymers share some properties with the structural components but may have quite distinct actions in the gut. All of these components give plants their structure and form. Their physical and chemical properties are dependent also on the age and growing conditions of the plant.

Structural (Insoluble) Fiber

Cellulose

Cellulose is the best known, most widely distributed, and most truly fibrous component. It is a long, unbranched glucose polymer of great molecular weight. It has crystalline features, but its linear, unbranched nature accounts for its fibrous properties.

Although the amount of cellulose in the plant cell wall varies, it is plentiful in bran and apple peel. The cell wall of the cotton seed contains approximately 95 percent cellulose, but most plant cell walls have between 15 percent to 40 percent. Human gut enzymes do not digest cellulose but intestinal bacteria may do so. This feature and the ability of cellulose to hold water and bind certain substances are believed to account for much of its importance in the human diet; but other factors may be important as well.

Lignin

The term *lignin* is derived from the Latin word for "wood." Lignin provides stiffness as plants age, and is 40 percent to 50 percent of the cell wall of wood. It is also found in cereals and potatoes. Unlike other components of dietary fiber, lignin is not a carbohydrate; it is insoluble and constitutes a major portion of crude fiber. Its principal importance to the fiber story appears to be its capacity to inhibit breakdown of cell-wall carbohydrate.

Hemicellulose

There are at least 250 branched hemicellulose polymers that contain a mixture of pentose and hexose sugars. Some are soluble. These amorphous substances form a matrix in which are meshed cellulose fibers. Hemicellulose comprises 15 percent to 30 percent of plant cell walls. The pentose-containing polysaccharides (many sugars linked together) that are found especially in bran hemicellulose have the greatest effect on fecal bulk. The bulking and laxative action of fiber is attributable to its water-holding capacity and the proliferation of colon bacteria which feed on it. The bacterial degradation of fiber to short-chain fatty acids may also be important.

Nonstructural (Soluble) Fiber

Pectins

Pectins are not fibrous at all, but rather tend to gel. They are polysaccharides comprising 1 percent to 4 percent of most cell walls but are more plentiful in the skins of citrus fruits, apples, and onions. Pectins are closely bound to other cell-wall constituents, and readily hold water outside the gut.

Plant Gums and Mucilages

Such substances as plant gums and mucilages are neither fibrous nor strictly confined to the cell wall. Like pectins, they have water-holding properties. They are not digested by small-gut enzymes, a fact that explains their inclusion as "dietary fiber."

Gums are sticky substances that seal plant wounds. Commercially, they are used as adhesives or as food additives. Some gums are bulk-forming laxatives, such as karaya gum and tragacanth, obtained from the stems and seeds of tropical plants. Guar gum is used as a thickener in salad dressing, toothpaste, and soups, and also is an ingredient in laxatives. Mucilages are hydrophilic substances that retain moisture for the seed. There are mucilages in psyllium that are believed responsible for the bulking and laxative properties of that widely used substance.

Algal Polysaccharides

Sometimes called mucilages, algal polysaccharides are uniquely found in the cell walls of algae and seaweed. The important one is agar, which has gel-forming and water-holding properties. These properties account for agar's ability to increase fecal bulk and explain its use in laxative preparations.

Other Substances in Dietary Fiber

There are a number of substances associated with dietary fiber that should be considered briefly. Phytate is present in the cell walls of most seeds and is of interest because of its ability to bind iron, calcium, magnesium, and zinc. Although whole wheat bread contains more iron than white bread, this mineral is better absorbed from the latter. Although there has been concern that fiber might impair absorption of these minerals, there is no evidence that this is clinically important. The waxy film on apples is an example of the cuticular substances that protect plants.

COLONIC FLORA

Our colons are populated by a variety of bacteria. Intestinal immunity adapts to this situation, and these organisms are allowed to coexist within us as long as they refrain from invading the mucosa. Ordinarily, the arrangement is of mutual benefit. As host, we provide heat, food, and shelter (not light), while our tenants mind their own business and prevent the overgrowth of intruders who might harm us both. Experience with germ-free animals confirms our interdependence. Raised under sterile conditions, such laboratory animals are miserable creatures indeed. Because these animals have no gut organisms to stimulate their immune system, antibody-producing cells are poorly developed and antibodies are deficient. The cecum of such an animal is thin-walled, distended, and sluggish. However, these abnormalities can be corrected by the presence of colon bacteria.

We tamper with our bacterial tenants at our peril. Acute diarrhea is frequently encountered during treatment with antibiotics, a phenomenon attributed to altered gut flora. In many instances, it is the enterotoxin-emitting *Clostridium difficile* bacteria which gains the upper hand (if bacteria have hands!). The diarrhea usually subsides when the drug is withdrawn, but occasionally a grave complication called pseudomembranous enterocolitis occurs.

The bacteria in the colon are many and varied. That they have important and complex interrelationships with dietary fiber, and that they are a substantial component of stool mass, will become apparent in the next section.

PHYSICAL PROPERTIES OF FIBER

Fiber in the plant cell wall can be visualized as a weave of linear molecules of cellulose enmeshing other structural components, such as lignin and hemicellulose. Nonstructural polysaccharides in the interstices have water-holding, gelling, and adhesive effects. Obviously, the nature of the structure depends upon the source of the fiber. Grass contains more protein and sugar in the spring than later in the year. Maturing plant stems contain progressively more lignin, which adds hardness to the cell wall. Thus, the physical and chemical properties of dietary fiber from plants of different maturity vary greatly.

The ability of fiber to hold water is believed an important determinant of stool weight and gastrointestinal transit time. Initially, water adsorbs to the surface of the fiber. More water fills in the interstices. The water-holding capacity of fiber ranges from 4.5 grams of water per gram of bran, and 2 grams of water per gram of carrot, to 0.4 grams of water per gram of potato. Water that exceeds this capacity is called *free water*. In diarrhea, free water exists in excess of the ability of dietary fiber to adsorb it. Fine bran has less water-holding capacity than coarse bran.

Dietary fiber is variably digested in human beings by colon bacteria. Cellulose, for example, is 50 percent digested but subject to many modifying factors. Reducing the particle size of coarse bran renders the cellulose (and other fibers) more accessible to bacteria. Thus, fine bran is more digested and less survives in feces.

Lignin is not broken down by bacteria and, through its physical relationship with cellulose, reduces the latter's susceptibility to bacterial degradation. Bran, one of the commonest lignified substances in the human diet, likely owes its effectiveness as a stool-bulking agent to lignin's resistance to bacterial degradation.

Although the bacterial digestion of cellulose proceeds rapidly in the first 12 hours, it continues for at least 24 hours. Thus, the time necessary for bran to transit the gut is an important consideration. The longer the transit time, the greater the fiber breakdown. Thus, a high-fiber diet, by reducing transit time, allows more intact fiber to appear in the stool, thus enhancing its local effect.

RESULTS OF FIBER BREAKDOWN

Fermentation of dietary fiber, whether it takes place in the rumen (stomach) of a cow, the cecum of a rodent, or the colon of a human being, results in three important products: volatile fatty acids (VFA), gas, and energy. The volatile fatty acids are acetate, propionate, and butyrate. They are important sources of energy for the cow or the rabbit, but much less so for human beings. They appear to have laxative properties as well.

Hydrogen, methane, and carbon dioxide are the important products of bacterial fermentation, which helps to explain why many people find a high-fiber diet an inflating experience, at least in the beginning (see Chapter 12). Many people avoid such a diet because it is gassy; yet the improved transit may paradoxically reduce the time available for fermentation and thus eventually reduce colon gas.

Finally, colonic bacteria use the energy released by their digestive activities to greatly increase their numbers. This has a significant effect on stool weight. Although feces are 70 percent to 80 percent water, the remaining solid is roughly half undigested fiber and half bacterial mass.

Undoubtedly, fiber has other intracolonic effects as well. By holding water, it may provide a local micro-environment that favors metabolic processes or protects certain solutes from bacterial attack. This is a fertile area for research.

THE EFFECT OF FIBER IN HUMAN BEINGS

The fate of nations depends upon how they are fed.

Anthelme Brillat-Savarin (1755–1826)

On Stool

For 50 years, bran has been known to expand and soften the stool. Cellulose and nondietary bulking agents, such as psyllium, are widely prescribed for constipation. In the previous section, we discussed how dietary fiber, such as that in bran, might increase fecal bulk. This bulking effect is dose-related in human beings. In a cereal, 11.2 grams of dietary fiber will increase the daily stool weight by 25 grams while 19 grams will cause a 55-gram increase. These amounts of dietary fiber correspond to a daily intake of 30 to 60 grams (2–4 tablespoonfuls) of Kellogg's All-Bran, respectively.

It should not be assumed that dietary fiber is the only determinant of stool weight. In one study, with dietary fiber held constant, larger stools were associated with strong ego and an outgoing personality. Thus, many local and environmental factors alter gut motility and secretion, probably through the enteric nervous system (see Chapter 7), and account for the great variability in stool weight.

Bran will hurry gastrointestinal transit in those in whom it is slow, and may slow it in those in whom it is fast. It appears that at least 20 grams of unprocessed bran are necessary each day to achieve an effect on transit. Coarse bran reduces transit time more than fine bran, perhaps because of its greater water-holding capacity or its resistance to bacterial degradation. Processing or cooking bran destroys much of its bulking and laxative activity.

Some fiber, as we have mentioned, is destroyed by gut bacteria. Pectin, although hydrophilic, is completely digested in the colon and therefore has no effect on fecal bulk. The increase in stool bulk induced by other fiber is greater than that of stool weight, perhaps owing to the trapping of gas. The proportion of water to solid in the stool changes little. Dietary fiber purified from great quantities of cabbage, carrot, apple, and guar gum had much less effect than bran fiber on stool weight and transit. The exact mechanism of fiber's bulking and laxative effects remains to be defined, and our understanding of feces composition remains rudimentary.

The use of dietary fiber, especially bran and psyllium, in the

Table 7
Fiber Content of Some Foods

Food	Size of serving	Fiber content per serving (grams)
Vegetables (cooked, unless otherwise noted)		
Asparagus	¾ cup	3.10
Bean sprouts, raw	½ cup	1.60
Beans		
Green	½ cup	2.10
Kidney	½ cup	5.80
Lima	½ cup	4.40
Pinto	½ cup	5.30
White	½ cup	5.00
Broccoli	½ cup	2.00
Brussels sprouts	½ cup	3.90
Cabbage	½ cup	2.00
Carrots	½ cup	2.30
Cauliflower	½ cup	1.60
Celery, raw	½ cup	1.30
Corn		
Cream, canned	½ cup	5.10
Kernels	½ cup	3.90
Eggplant	½ cup	2.00
Lettuce, raw	½ cup	0.30
Onions, raw	½ cup	2.60
Peas	½ cup	4.10
Potatoes		
Sweet, baked	½ large	1.70
White, baked	½ medium	1.90
Radishes, raw	5 medium	0.60
Squash		
Acorn	½ cup	4.30
Zucchini	½ cup	2.70
Tomatoes, raw	1 medium	0.80
Turnips	½ cup	1.70
Fruits (raw)		
Apple, with skin	1	2.80
Apricots	2	1.50

(continued)

Table 7 (*continued*)

Food	Size of serving	Fiber content per serving (grams)
	Fruits (raw)	
Banana	½ medium	1.00
Blackberries	½ cup	4.50
Cherries	10	1.20
Grapefruit	½ medium	1.70
Grapes	12	0.50
Orange	1 small	1.20
Peach	1 medium	1.60
Pear	½ medium	2.50
Pineapple	½ cup	1.20
Plums	3 small	1.80
Raspberries	¾ cup	6.80
Strawberries	¾ cup	2.00
	Grain and other products	
Bread		
French	1 slice	1.00
Rye	1 slice	0.90
White enriched	1 slice	0.50
Whole wheat	1 slice	1.40
Cereal		
All-Bran (100%)	⅓ cup	8.60
Corn Flakes	1 cup	0.40
Shredded Wheat	1 biscuit	2.80
Wheaties	1 cup	2.60
Crackers		
Graham	2 squares	2.80
Saltine	6 crackers	0.70
Rice		
Brown	½ cup	2.40
White	½ cup	0.10
Spaghetti	½ cup	0.80
Almonds	1 tbsp	1.10

treatment of the irritable gut will be discussed in Chapters 13, 16, and 19. The fiber content of some foods is shown in Table 7.

On Bile Acids

Dietary fiber alters the colonic handling of bile acids so that their concentration in the bile is increased. This, in turn, improves the solubility of cholesterol in the bile. These observations support the notion originally proposed by Cleave that a low-fiber diet reduces gall bladder bile acids and favors the development of cholesterol gallstones.

On Lipids

Some of the soluble or nonstructural components of fiber reduce serum cholesterol, but bran is ineffective. The doses of pectin or guar gum required to reduce cholesterol are too large to be practical.

On Nutrition

Increased dietary fiber intake leads to increased short-term loss of fat, nitrogen, calcium, iron, and zinc in the feces. It is interesting to note, in this connection, that among the defenders during the seige of Kut (Iraq) in 1915, many British troops acquired beriberi, whereas no Indian soldiers succumbed. It is believed that whole wheat chapaties provided the necessary vitamin B_1 that protected the Indians. Thus, the nutritional implications of fiber for patients who are encouraged to eat large doses of bran require more research.

With reasonable doses of dietary fiber intake, there is little risk of mineral deficiency. However, rickets and osteomalacia occur in the Middle East and in India where 70 percent or more of body energy is provided by whole wheat bread or chapaties. Similarly,

zinc and iron deficiency might occur in susceptible people on a
very high-fiber diet.

On Diabetes and Obesity

Pectin and guar gum, the gel-forming polysaccharides, improve oral glucose (sugar) tolerance, lessen urine sugar, and reduce
insulin output in diabetics. In adult-onset diabetics, a high-car-
bohydrate diet with 15 or 20 grams of crude fiber reduces the need
for insulin. Pectin and guar reduce the reactive hypoglycemia (low
blood sugar) of patients who have had part of their stomach removed for ulcer. These effects appear to be due to increased vis-
cosity of gut contents, which slows transit in the upper gut and
delays sugar absorption.

High-fiber diets may limit energy intake. They are filling, are
less energy dense, and may reduce fat absorption. The fiber of
whole apples compared to apple juice of the same energy content
increases satiety, improves glucose tolerance, and lowers insulin
demand. Whole wheat bread produces satiety with less caloric intake than white bread. Normal subjects take an average of 45 minutes to chew and swallow 300 grams of whole wheat bread,
whereas they devour the same amount of white bread in 34 minutes. Thus, to gain weight on whole wheat bread requires more
effort. This evidence favors Cleave's theory that diabetes and obesity result from diets rich in refined carbohydrates.

On Protection of the Gut

Finally, fiber may protect us. In an experiment, sodium cycla-
mate administered in a dose that was lethal to rats who were on
a purified diet was harmless in the rats who were fed a high-fiber
diet. Rats on a high-fiber diet were also apparently protected from
the colon cancer-inducing activity of some substances (carcinogens). By diluting and expediting transit of possible carcinogens,
fiber might prevent colon cancer in humans. Also, rats fed a low-

residue diet develop diverticular disease, which can be prevented by a bulky diet or by psyllium. This beneficial effect of fiber has not yet been proven in human beings (see Chapter 19). Despite the above data, fiber deficiency is not proved to be the cause of serious human colon disease. Even if it were, experience with the antitobacco campaign suggests that bringing this knowledge to bear on the population would be difficult.

It is possible that fiber deficiency is important in the genesis of many functional bowel complaints. Meanwhile, most gastroenterologists recommend dietary fiber in the management of constipation and the irritable bowel syndrome.

SUMMARY

The fiber hypothesis suggests that the removal of dietary fiber from the diet by food processing is responsible for many of the gut diseases of Western populations. Included among these are carcinoma of the colon, diverticular disease, the irritable bowel, and possibly other syndromes of the irritable gut. Dietary fiber is derived from plant cell walls and consists of cellulose, hemicellulose, lignin, and a number of soluble substances, such as pectins, gums, and mucilages. These components differ greatly in their chemical and physical properties and in their effects on the gut. A diet that contains a large amount of wheat bran tends to produce a larger stool and more rapid transit through the gastrointestinal tract. Clinical studies of these effects support the notion that a high-fiber diet is useful in most types of constipation. The use of a high-fiber diet in the irritable bowel is less well substantiated.

Meanwhile, it is important to know that dietary fiber with its complex interrelationships with the intestinal flora may influence the metabolism of bile acids, lipids, and other nutrients, and may have a role to play in the prevention and treatment of diabetes and obesity.

The extent of interaction of fiber with bacteria, bile salts, toxins, minerals, and carcinogens is just beginning to be appreciated. Clearly, bran has improved its image since Shakespeare wrote:

> . . . he would mouth with a beggar though she smelt brown bread and garlic.

Measure for Measure (3.2)

CHAPTER SEVEN

Gut Reactions
The Mind–Gut Axis

Man may inherit a sick, irritable nervous system, another may spoil a good one with bad habits or bad training, or a good one may be shocked out of action by the blows of circumstance.

Sir William Osler

The gut often provides an outlet for the emotions. The relationship of soma to psyche is perhaps greater than many will admit, even though it is apparent that our guts react to events in our environment. Who has escaped the queasy stomach or the loose bowels that often accompany stressful ventures? Such "gut feelings" may occur in a variety of situations: at a board meeting, during an examination, or at a hockey game. The effect of emotion on gut function, however profound, is unpredictable. When soldiers are ordered into battle, for example, some are nauseated, some vomit, some are incontinent, and some experience a curious sense of well-being—a release at the prospect of action. It is a common experience that contemplation of a difficult situation may elicit more gut reaction than the situation itself.

EFFECT OF EMOTION ON GUT FUNCTION

Normally, the gut works silently, accepting whatever we feed it and seldom intruding into our consciousness except to signal hunger, satiety, and the need to defecate. Its silent workings are governed by the enteric nervous system (ENS) with its complex network of nerves, hormones, and neurotransmitter substances. In Chapter 1, we saw that the ENS, or "gut brain," is intricately connected with the central nervous system or brain (Figure 3). Thus, the mechanisms are in place for the brain to sense events in the gut and to alter gut function. Many famous physiologists have studied the effects of emotion on the gut, and it is pertinent to review some of their observations.

Stomach Reaction

The science of gut reaction began in 1833 with the observations of William Beaumont, a surgeon in the U.S. Army. Alexis St. Martin, a French Canadian voyageur, had suffered an accidental gunshot wound in the abdomen which resulted in a gastric fistula, that is, an opening of the stomach to the abdominal wall. Beaumont cared for St. Martin under frontier conditions for many years and recorded his observations. When St. Martin experienced fear, anger, or impatience, his stomach mucosa could be seen through the fistula to become pale and to produce less gastric juice. In 1928, Dr. F. Hoetzel of Chicago sampled, in the interest of science, his own gastric juice each morning by means of a tube. Contrary to St. Martin, he noted that his gastric-acid secretion increased when his landlady was shot during a robbery and remained high while his fear of gangsters persisted. Perhaps Hoetzel had the tough viscera necessary for survival in Al Capone's Chicago! In other studies, both increased and decreased gastric-acid secretion are observed in response to strong emotion. In their gastric fistula patient "Tom," the American scientists Wolf and Wolff noted increased gastric vascularity (blushing), secretion and movement in response to hostility, and resentment and anxiety, whereas the opposite occurred in response to fear and sadness. When the gastric mucosa blushes, the threshold for pain induced by distension of a balloon within the stomach is lowered. Tom may have had a personality that favored such specific reactions. Perhaps a person's stomach learns to respond to certain situations in a highly individual way just as Pavlov's dog learned to salivate in response to a bell. Thus, the stomach may be a window to the emotions, but it is paned with fluted glass.

A further glimpse at the complexities of gastrointestinal reactivity is afforded by the executive monkey experiment. Two monkeys, tied side by side, received electric shocks at irregular intervals, but only one—"the executive"—was able to arrest the shock once it started. He learned to do this by pressing a button at the side of his chair. Constant vigilance was required to control his fate and, incidentally, that of his companion. The second monkey did not have access to a button and became resigned to his lot. Duodenal ulcers developed exclusively in the executive, proving that, at least in monkeys, fatalism is healthy.

Rats appear more suited to the executive role. In a series of experiments, rats were placed in restraint cages, a situation known to cause gastric erosions. Rats 1 and 2 received electric shocks, whereas only rat 1 could prevent the shock when warned by a buzzer. In this case, rat 1, the executive, was less likely to suffer an ulcer than rat 2, which could not control its frustrating situation. The response of these rats could be modified by developmental factors. For example, handling the animals prior to weaning made them less susceptible to the ulcerogenic effects of restraints when they became adults. Rats that were reared alone were more resistant to the effects of restraint than their fellows raised in groups.

With regard to human beings, I. A. Mirsky suggested that to precipitate a duodenal ulcer, there must be (1) a physiologically susceptible person, say, a hypersecretor of gastric acid; (2) psychological conflicts; and (3) an environment noxious to the individual. To test this hypothesis, he selected 2 groups of U.S. Army draftees. One group consisted of gastric-pepsinogen hypersecretors. Four of the 63 hypersecretors had duodenal ulcer upon induction, and 5 more developed one during a 16-week training period. No ulcer occurred in those individuals secreting normal amounts of pepsinogen. Mirsky suggested that the hypersecretors who were thrust into the hostile environment of the army experienced conflict between their emotional need and its gratification, a notion beyond the sympathies of the average drill sergeant.

Gastric secretion increases in response to a stressful interview. This may arise in the hypothalamus of the brain and may affect the stomach either through the vagus nerve or through hormones released by the pituitary gland. Such a response can be conditioned so that acid secretion increases with the mere appearance of the interviewer. A cerebral effect on gastric secretion is further demonstrated by research from Argentina. In an experiment, young men increased their stomach-acid output while reading erotic literature. Like politics, love is risky in Argentina.

Much has been made of these experiments in considering the etiology of peptic ulcers. What concerns us here is that emotion may affect gastric function. The effects of *chronic* emotion or stress on gastric motility and secretion are not precisely known, but there can be little doubt that they are important in the genesis of symptoms. For example, emotion may precipitate the gastric dysfunction that we think accompanies some cases of nonulcer dyspepsia. Thus, a certain personality type with certain previous experiences and associations may undergo changes in gastric function or in awareness of gastric function in response to emotion.

Colon Reaction

In 1909, Walter Cannon observed that when a cat is stressed, its entire gut relaxes except the sigmoid. Yet it was over a century after Beaumont peered into St. Martin's stomach before a researcher actually gazed at the colon under experimental conditions. Almy and his associates (1950) conducted a series of experiments designed to illustrate the effect of emotion on the colon. Observations on healthy young medical students included sigmoidoscopic estimation of lumen diameter, vascularity (blushing), secretion, and sigmoid pressure recording. Stress was induced by painful immersion of the hand in ice water, a screw-tightened headband, hypoglycemia, and an "unsympathetic" interview.

The painful stimuli led to blushing, increased pressure, and hypersecretion of the sigmoid colon. First, the pain was perceived and then the emotional conflict was noted (Why did I get involved with this?). It was the conflict that caused the colon reaction. As with Cannon's cats, sigmoid tone increased. In one experiment, a medical student volunteered to have his sigmoid colon studied through a sigmoidoscope. During the procedure, one of the researchers mentioned cancer of the colon, leading the student to believe he had one. At that point, the mucosal lining of the bowel was observed to blush and contract vigorously. When the student was reassured that no cancer existed, his colon resumed its normal pallor and relaxed. (We trust that the student graduated successfully.)

In another experiment, Almy (1950) measured colon pressure in a woman during a stressful interview. When the subject was saddened or tearful during the interview, colon pressure fell; when she was made angry, colon pressure increased. Although this experiment suggests a new meaning for the word *uptight*, it cannot be predicted that exactly similar reactions will occur in all persons, or even in the same person at different times. There is no doubt, however, that stress can alter gut function. Almy postulated that in times of combat, primeval reflexes relax upper gastrointestinal activity to preserve the body economy for action. The sigmoid contracts to prevent embarrassing loss of feces—a consideration that might have been crucial in a medieval suit of armor. It is the individual's perception of a threat to his security that leads to this reaction. The headscrew, painful in a vital part but not dangerous, produced sigmoid reaction, whereas hypoglycemia, potentially more dangerous, did not. Repeated application of the same stress was less likely to affect colon function because the subjects were no longer frightened by it. Almy (1950) concluded that in patients with the irritable bowel, the disorder is "not in the bowel but in the environment, and in the patient's attitude towards his environment."

Other Gut Reactions

Lest the reader think that only the stomach and colon react to emotion, we should acknowledge the small-bowel experiments of David Wingate (McRae et al., 1982). Using a sophisticated radio device anchored in the small bowel, Wingate recorded pressure waves in response to various stimuli. Individuals with this device in place were required to drive in London traffic, read into a microphone which delayed the sound playback, play frustrating video games, and be awakened by loud noises in the night. Not surprisingly, he found that such stimuli altered small-intestinal movements, and some of his data suggest that this alteration is more marked or different in patients with the irritable bowel syndrome (IBS). Others have noted altered small-gut secretion in IBS patients. It seems likely that the small gut is as important a player in the irritable gut as the colon.

Stressful interviews can induce nonpropulsive contractions of the lower esophagus. Emotional reaction is also believed to be involved in globus, esophageal spasm, and heartburn, but studies such as those of the stomach and colon are nonexistent. It is possible to conclude, however, that all segments of the gut may react to emotional stress.

EFFECT OF THE GUT ON EMOTION

We must not consider the nervous connections between the brain and the gut as a one-way street. In fact, there is more traffic from the gut to the brain than vice versa. It is evident that a diseased gut sends signals to the brain, and that these signals may have a profound effect on emotion and behavior. The gut and the mind are clearly linked.

In Chapters 13 and 14, the mechanism of functional abdominal pain will be discussed. Balloons inflated at certain sites within the gut lumen can reproduce the abdominal pain of most IBS patients (Figure 23). This procedure seems to confirm the gut as the site of origin for the pain. It does not establish, however, whether the pain is due to a local gut abnormality, such as spasm, or whether the sufferer is abnormally aware of a normal event in the gut. In some cases, it seems likely that both events are at work. Could, for example, a person whose parent dies of colon cancer suddenly become morbidly aware of a mild cramp that has existed subconsciously for years?

Functional gut disease often coexists with depression, prompting the questions which came first and did one cause the other. Patients usually believe that the gut symptoms cause the depression, but this most likely reflects public attitudes toward mental as opposed to physical illness. Many psychiatrists believe that depression, or other mental disorder, causes the somatic symptoms and, in some people, this may be the case. They cite numerous studies showing that IBS or other functional gut disease patients have more psychiatric or personality disorders than those with organic bowel disease or normal controls. The faulty methodology of these studies is discussed by Creed and Guthrie. Of importance here is the observation that IBS patients in these studies are a special subgroup of all IBS sufferers. First, they are part of the minority of patients who see physicians for IBS symptoms. Second, they are referred to a center that is interested in such studies. Third, they submit themselves to a research protocol. Two recent reports have exposed the fallacy of such studies. In separate observations, Drossman (1988) and Whitehead (1988) showed that IBS sufferers who do *not* see doctors have personality or psychological profiles similar to asymptomatic nonpatients. Could it be that when IBS and a psychological or personality disorder occur together, it is the latter that interferes with the patient's ability to cope with the symptoms and triggers the consultation?

ILLNESS BEHAVIOR

From the foregoing discussion it can be seen that reporting irritable gut symptoms to a doctor is a critical act. A person with functional symptoms that might be ignored by most sufferers now becomes a patient, and may therefore expose himself to investigations and treatments which may not be beneficial. Why has this decision been made? Severity of symptoms may be an easy answer, but many observers suspect it is not the correct one. In many patients, health-seeking or illness behavior appears to be important.

Through random telephone interviews in Cincinnati, Whitehead discovered that sufferers of IBS symptoms, when compared to those with organic gut disease, were more likely to have received favors when ill as a child, to regard colds more seriously, and to consult a doctor for minor complaints. This concept of illness behavior makes the IBS patient more understandable and underlines the mind–body integration of human disease. Whether or not gut or psychological symptoms cause each other, they both certainly contribute to the way in which the sufferer interprets and reacts to the symptoms.

Thus, a person with IBS symptoms may go to a doctor because that's the way he learned to react to symptoms as a child, or because he has a personality or emotional disorder. In our society, emotional disturbances are not socially acceptable, and anxious or depressed people may use IBS symptoms as a front to legitimize their underlying emotional distress. It is also becoming clear that a previously well person may begin to suffer IBS or dyspeptic symptoms, or at least report them to a doctor, after a stressful life-event (see below). This illness behavior is so much a part of current thinking of the IBS that some observers suggest that it be included in the definition. Thus, gut symptoms do not constitute the IBS unless the sufferer consults. The philosophical question posed here is, do IBS symptoms unobserved in the population, like trees falling in the forest, really occur? Certainly, it is the reporting of the IBS to the doctor that creates the medical problem.

STRESSFUL LIFE EVENTS

Studies conducted in Britain indicate that clinic patients with IBS and dyspepsia are more likely than those with organic disease to have had a serious, threatening life-event in the 6 to 9 months prior to their visit. Usually, these events concern loss of a job, a family breakup, or serious illness or death in the family. Among patients undergoing appendectomy, those whose appendix turned out to be normal were more likely than the others to have had such a threatening life-event prior to surgery and to continue to be symptomatic a year later. It has even been observed that symptoms of a particular kind often follow publicity given to an illness of a well-known personality, as for example the colonic polyps of former President Reagan.

It is debatable whether these events cause the symptoms or make previously ignored symptoms important, thereby precipitating medical consultation. In either case, these events cannot be ignored, and may be the most important clue to management. A man who has just lost a father from colon cancer may merely require reassurance that his cramps or gas do not represent the same process. Of course, other situations are more complex.

PSYCHIATRIC ENTITIES AND PSYCHODYNAMICS

There is no doubt that some IBS patients may have a neurosis or psychosis, but a detailed discussion of these patients here is inappropriate. The complex interrelationships between soma and psyche have puzzled gastroenterologists for most of this century (Thompson, 1979). Fifty years ago, Walter Alverez used such terms as "over-taxed nervous system" and "constitutional inadequacy" and concluded "that there are a large number of dyspeptics who appear to have been born to be dyspeptic all their days." He despaired of curing them. Another physician stated that "in consulting a doctor, this type of patient hopes to justify his solution—getting sick—for his problem. The job of a doctor is to find a less incapacitating answer." Often this is a tall order! One early twentieth-century physician described some IBS patients who "belong to the hapless group of bed-ridden invalids dwelling on their illness, interested in their motions, and apparently almost loving their complaint." Robert Hutchison called such a patient "the abdominal woman" (see Chapter 14).

Most of these descriptions tell us more about the frustration of physicians than the cause of the patient's complaints, but they do serve to illustrate one extreme of the irritable gut. Attempts have been made to explain such symptoms as constipation or pain as atonement for guilt, or as the consequence of sexual repression, but little practical therapeutic benefit has resulted. (In Chapter 14, we will describe the pain-prone patient and provide a brief discussion of hypochondriasis and hysteria.)

Another condition to be considered is somatization disorder. It occurs almost exclusively in women, and is a chronic relapsing disorder manifested by recurrent multisystem symptoms without organic disease. The diagnosis is made in women who have at least 14 of 37 possible unexplained symptoms in many diverse organs, each of which has resulted in medication, alteration of life pattern, or a visit to the doctor. Since these patient's lives revolve around their chronic symptoms, the best treatment approach is a sound, long-term doctor–patient relationship without medication or repeated tests.

COMMENT

Although great advances in biomedical science have been made in the last 175 years, they have not been matched by an understanding of how emotion affects the body. Consequently, much of our belief about the role of the psyche in the pathogenesis of disease rests on unsubstantiated anecdotes or the uncontrolled study of behavioral therapy in patients with undecided illnesses.

In a subject so bereft of fact and yet so brimming with conflicting beliefs, there can be no recognized universal truth. The science of functional disorders is in a state similar to that of the science of bacteriology a century ago. Engel pointed out that such terms as stress, tension, anxiety, and emotional upset are as imprecise and diagnostically or therapeutically unhelpful as were the words catarrh, fever, or dropsy in bygone days. How does disturbed emotion disturb the gut? Perhaps what is needed is another Robert Koch or Louis Pasteur to lead us to an understanding of the nature of functional disease.

PART TWO

Gut Reactions

Syndromes of the Irritable Gut

CHAPTER EIGHT

Globus
A Lump in the Throat

The Globus hystericus is a spasmodic affection, sometimes appearing wholly in the pharynx.

Caleb Parry (1815)

Nearly one half of 147 adults who were interviewed in Bristol, England, recalled experiencing a "lump" in the throat. This particular sensation accounts for 3 percent of consultations to throat specialists. Indeed, it may be a normal sensation that is experienced by almost everybody at sometime in his or her life.

CLINICAL DESCRIPTION

Globus is Latin for "globe" or "ball." Typically, the subject describes a lump or ball in the throat at the level of the Adam's apple. Among the 147 young and middle-aged subjects who said they experienced a lump in the throat, only 3 percent related it to meals (Table 8). Seventy-five percent said that it occurred between meals. There was a similar prevalence in men and women, which

93

Table 8
Presence of Globus in 67 Subjects[a]

Feature	Subjects reporting (%)
Related to eating	3
Between meals	75
Related to strong emotion	96
Improved with swallow	19
Worse with swallow	9

[a] Adapted from *Canadian Medical Association Journal* (1982;126:46–48).

belies the alleged occurrence of globus in young, neurotic females. Almost all subjects said that the sensation occurred with strong emotion, and many volunteered that it disappeared when they cried. About one fifth of the patients claimed they were relieved if they swallowed, whereas one in ten felt that swallowing made it worse. Globus is unassociated with true dysphagia, pain, or weight loss. Some individuals consider the symptom to be, like tears, part of their emotional life.

It is suggested that globus occurs more frequently in individuals with the irritable bowel syndrome than others. However, in the 147 subjects described above, IBS symptoms were no more common in those with globus than in those without; neither did there seem to be any relationship between globus and heartburn. Reported associations with abnormalities of the cervical spine or with hiatus hernia are likely coincidental.

CAUSE

A Motor Disorder

One experienced radiologist, R. Schatzki, suggests that tense people swallow repeatedly, perhaps suffering from the dry mouth that accompanies anxiety. He claims that the symptom may be reproduced at will by repeated dry swallows. As the individual runs out of saliva, he becomes aware that he can no longer swallow and experiences a lump in the throat. The sensation, unlike true difficulty in swallowing, is sometimes relieved by taking food or drink.

A small number of globus patients are said to have a radiologically demonstrable hyperactive cricopharyngeal muscle or upper esophageal sphincter (UES) (see Figure 4). In one study, elevated UES pressures were recorded in 9 globus patients. In another report, UES contraction intervals were shortened while pharyngeal contraction intervals were prolonged in globus subjects. The UES pressure increases with the presence of fluid or acid in the esophagus. Perhaps upper sphincter contraction is triggered by gastroesophageal reflux in order to protect the respiratory passage. However, a recent study indicates no difference in UES pressure between small numbers of normals and patients with heartburn and globus. As mentioned, heartburn and globus do not necessarily occur together. Thus, it remains unsettled whether UES dysfunction is responsible for the globus sensation.

An Emotional Disorder

It brings a lump to the throat.

Anonymous

"It is a callous kid indeed who has never experienced momentary globus hystericus during a sad movie." Thus did the prominent physician E. D. Palmer (1967) recognize that globus is commonplace and related to emotion. People become "choked up" with grief or disappointment, and in some it may become a chronic, troublesome problem.

Advocates of psychosomatics such as George Engel (1977) say globus results from increased cricopharyngeal tension caused by inhibited crying. They speculate that crying and hunger are intimately associated developmentally. Suppression of crying in later life may represent unwillingness to accept a loss. This action simultaneously "evokes conflicting impulses to swallow and regurgitate, physiologically reflected in cricopharyngeal spasm, and symptomatically felt as a lump in the throat" (Glaser and Engel, 1977). Crying may bring emotional and symptomatic relief.

This hypothesis need not be swallowed whole! Suffice it to say that the globus sensation may be due to contraction of the throat muscles, which, in turn, may be initiated by emotion. This emotion need not be grief. A lump in the throat may be evoked by thoughts of home (nostalgia), the national anthem (pride), or an imminent reunion (love). As with the other disorders of the irritable gut, globus appears to occur in persons with an exceptionally responsive or sensitive gut wall, in this case, the cricopharyngeal muscle or UES. Such a response, occurring in nearly half of adults, must be natural and must not be caused by perverted emotional development. The epithet "hystericus" is traditionally added to "globus," but this is unfair. In a series of 231 patients with globus, hysteria was not a predominant feature.

DIAGNOSIS

The hysteric globe in the throat is scarcely ever heard of among men, but is one of the most familiar symptoms with hysteric women.

William Heberden (1710–1801)
Commentaries on the History and Cure of Diseases

Contrary to what is traditionally believed, globus is neither confined to women nor associated with hysteria. Persons with globus experience a lump in the throat and/or transient difficulty in swallowing *between* meals. Unlike patients with organic dysphagia (difficulty swallowing food), globus sufferers are often relieved by food, drink, or tears. Pain and weight loss are not features of globus, but attacks may be related to tension or emotion. Therefore, the presence or absence of these features should be ascertained by careful attention to the description of the symptom. True dysphagia is probably never functional, although diffuse esophageal spasm is a possible exception (see Chapter 9). When uncertain if the patient has dysphagia or globus, the prudent physician will order a barium x-ray of the esophagus or an endoscopy to exclude stricture and cancer (see Chapter 22).

Since the pathophysiology of globus is unknown, esophageal manometry (intraluminal pressure recording) seems an unnecessary frill with no therapeutic implications. Once the x-ray or endoscopy is done, the physician and the patient should be reassured without the need for other tests, which are unpleasant and may reinforce fear of organic disease.

TREATMENT

As is true with other manifestations of the irritable gut, a sympathetic hearing, careful physical examination, explanation, and reassurance constitute the foundations of therapy. The patient is entitled to believe that serious illness has been excluded. In the absence of any controlled trial, we must rely on anecdotal reports that the opportunity to discuss painful memories may relieve symptoms. Many patients say they are relieved from an episode of globus only when they submit themselves to a good cry. Sufferers must deal with underlying depression, grief, or anxiety. Beyond that, the physician should surely avoid prescribing drugs for this benign, recurrent, inconsequential symptom, which is so prevalent in the population.

SUMMARY

Globus, the feeling that there is a "ball" or "lump" in the throat, occurs in half of all adults. Often this sensation is associated with grief, anxiety, or other strong emotion, and can possibly be an indication of an abnormally sensitive or reactive upper esophageal sphincter. Globus is unrelated to the irritable bowel or heartburn. It occurs independently of eating and may improve with the swallowing of food or drink. Usually it disappears with crying. Like tears, it may need no psychodynamic explanation, but rather may reflect the quality or quantity of emotion. When repetitive and disabling, globus may indicate an abnormal emotional state. Careful attention to historical details of the symptom will allow the physician to distinguish globus from dysphagia. In doubtful cases, endoscopy or x-ray of the esophagus is indicated to ensure that no stricture or cancer exists. Satisfactory management depends upon the patient's confidence in the physician's explanation and a sympathetic discussion of associated emotions.

CHAPTER NINE

The Irritable Esophagus

When an individual develops chest pain, he or she is normally referred to a cardiologist. However, among such sufferers investigated for coronary artery disease, 10 percent to 30 percent are found to have normal coronary arteriograms (x-rays of the coronary arteries). Although a few of these sufferers are thought to have abnormalities of microscopic blood vessels in the heart, most are said to have "noncardiac chest pain." In the United States, individual sufferers with continuing chest pain spend an estimated $3,500 annually for doctor visits, drugs, and hospitalization.

What else is there in the chest to cause chest pain? Lungs are insensitive. Although inflammation of the outer lining of the lungs causes pleurisy, the pain is characteristic and is seldom confused with the discomfort that is due to coronary artery disease. Likewise, diseases of the bones, muscles, joints, and ligaments of the chest wall might be painful, but the pain is distinct from angina, and the affected parts are tender to touch. Thus, the esophagus becomes the scapegoat, and esophageal "spasm" the explanation.

As we shall see, science has not been very helpful in establishing the esophagus as the seat of chest pain. Before proceeding with the discussion, however, I wish to separate the esophageal motility disorders that cause pain from the reflux of gastric contents into the esophagus causing heartburn. Heartburn is a very com-

99

mon and precise syndrome and usually can be clearly identified by the patient and by the patient's description. Occasionally, there may be confusion of heartburn with cardiac pain, and some researchers believe that gastroesophageal reflux may sometimes trigger esophageal spasm. Heartburn and gastroesophageal reflux disease (GERD) will be dealt with in Chapter 10. Only noncardiac chest pain thought to be due to disturbed motility of the body of the esophagus will be discussed as the irritable esophagus.

MECHANISMS OF NONCARDIAC CHEST PAIN

In cardiac units, when coronary artery studies fail to demonstrate disease in a patient with chest pain, it is necessary to turn to the gastroenterologist to help pin it on the gullet. Through pressure sensors stationed within the esophagus, it is possible to record contractions and sphincter tone (see Figure 12). In most cases, such esophageal motility studies fail to prove that chest pain is due to the esophagus; and the presence of abnormalities in motility does not settle the issue, especially if the abnormality does not occur in unison with the pain. In a recent study (Richter et al., 1989), 24 patients with noncardiac chest pain wore intraesophageal devices for 24 hours that recorded motility disturbances and gastroesophageal reflux events (see description of the method below). Of 92 episodes of chest pain in these 24 individuals, only 20 percent coincided with reflux events, 12 percent with abnormal motility and 4 percent (1 patient) with both. Fully 64 percent of pains were accompanied by no recorded abnormality. Even in the case of those pains with associated abnormalities, the timing was inexact. Similar results have been found by others.

Several esophageal motor disturbances have been blamed for chest pain. The *nutcracker esophagus* is the most commonly recognized. In this disturbance, peristalsis is intact, but the pressure generated by the wave is greatly exaggerated and lasts longer. Some researchers believe that the nutcracker esophagus may become *diffuse esophageal spasm,* in which there are repetitive, nonperistaltic, high-pressure contractions (see Figure 13). These ab-

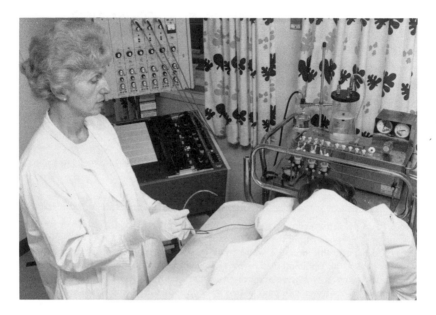

Figure 12. Esophageal motility. The nurse places a thin tube containing 3 recording catheters with tips sited at 5-centimeter intervals into the patient's esophagus (see text). The catheters are steadily perfused with water from the pump shown at right, and intraesophageal pressures are recorded by the electronic device to the left.

normalities may occur with or without chest pain, and the question whether they have anything to do with each other is moot. The latter pattern may be seen in the early stages of *achalasia*, a disease of esophageal denervation in which the lower esophageal sphincter (LES) will not relax, thus causing difficulty in swallowing (dysphagia). These abnormalities are difficult enough to correlate with chest pain, but what is the physician to make of decreased peristalsis, abnormal wave forms, occasional spontaneous or simultaneous contractions, or a hypertensive LES?

Against this weak evidence for esophageal spasm as a frequent cause of chest pain must be considered the notion of increased esophageal sensitivity. We do not know how esophageal pain is mediated, but it is believed that there are mechanoreceptors in the

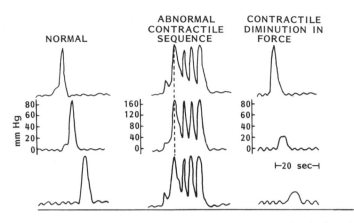

Figure 13. A pressure recording resulting from three pressure-sensing devices sited at 5-centimeter intervals within the esophagus. On the left is shown a normal, sequential passage of a peristaltic pressure wave over these sensors from top to bottom. The pressure peak is 80 millimeters of mercury. The center recordings illustrate simultaneous, repetitive waves generating pressures of 160 millimeters of mercury. When such "spasm" is observed with pain, it may be concluded that esophageal spasm is the cause, but such is the exception. The recordings on the right show one of the many other motility disturbances whose relationship to chest pain is very obscure.

intramuscular (myenteric) nerve plexes that transmit variations of esophageal tension through nerves to the central nervous system (Figure 3). We have already seen in Chapter 2 that balloon distension of the esophagus will stimulate contraction above and relaxation below. Sir Arthur Hurst, the famous British physiologist, demonstrated that balloon distension within the esophagus caused chest pain that radiated through to the back. Researchers at the Bowman Gray School of Medicine, North Carolina, recently used balloon distension to reproduce noncardiac chest pain in 56 percent of 50 patients (Richter et al., 1989). This was achieved at a lower pressure than that required to produce chest pain in 20 percent of 30 normal individuals. These results recall earlier studies in which pain of the irritable bowel was reproduced by intraintestinal balloon inflation (see Chapter 13).

Intraesophageal balloon distension is a new, provocative test for esophageal chest pain. More importantly, its results raise the question as to what extent is esophageal chest pain due to altered perception of normal esophageal motility rather than normal perception of altered esophageal motility? In many cases esophageal pain may not be a motor disorder at all.

PSYCHOLOGICAL FACTORS

It has long been suspected that there is a relationship of esophageal irritability to stress. As stated in Chapter 2, esophageal nonpropulsive or "tertiary" contractions increase with age. A century ago, it was observed that cold, hot, or carbonated drinks evoked such contractions. Even a loud noise, such as clapping the hands, elicits asymptomatic tertiary contractions. In contrast, a recent study has shown that a cold drink brings about transient paralysis of the esophagus, and it is suggested that the associated chest pain may be due to esophageal distension (see balloon data above).

Emotionally stressful interviews induce nonpropulsive contractions of the lower esophagus of normal persons. In one study of 50 patients referred for esophageal manometry, 25 had one or more of the following: increased amplitude of contraction, increased wave duration, or increased abnormal responses and triple-peaked waves. Of those with abnormal tracings, 83 percent had evidence of depression, anxiety, or somatization disorders according to established criteria, compared to 32 percent of the 25 without the abnormalities. The conclusion was that emotion may alter esophageal function as measured by manometry, but it is most uncertain how this alteration translates into symptoms. Another group observed that psychologic stress (difficult cognitive problems) caused increased lower esophageal contractions and generated anxiety in persons with noncardiac chest pain. These responses were greater than those of controls. Other researchers have linked continued noncardiac chest pain to hypochondriasis.

CLINICAL PRESENTATION

From the descriptions of sufferers, it is often not possible to distinguish cardiac pain from that thought to be due to the esophagus. It is not infrequent that a physician suspects both cardiac (angina) and noncardiac chest pain in the same patient. Both pains may be "squeezing," "tight," or "pressurelike" in nature. Nonetheless, pain that radiates to the arms and occurs with exertion is more likely to be cardiac. Pain radiating to the abdomen or back is probably esophageal, especially if provoked by meals or accompanied by difficulty in swallowing. The overlap is such, however, that distinction should not be made without x-rays of the coronary arteries. Even nitroglycerin, which is used for angina, may relieve noncardiac chest pain, and so may not be used to distinguish one pain from another.

Usually heartburn can be distinguished from the irritable esophagus by its relationship to meals and by its worsening with bending, straining, or reclining. Chest pain may be due to injury (bruises or fractured ribs) or to inflammation of joints where the ribs meet the sternum (breastbone), and of the joints of the sternum itself. Pleurisy and pericarditis are short illnesses that cause a sharp pain aggravated by breathing or coughing.

DIAGNOSIS

The investigation of someone complaining of chest pain, after cardiac and other causes have been excluded, should begin with a barium contrast x-ray of the esophagus. This procedure will exclude most mechanical causes, such as cancer or stricture (narrowing). If esophagitis is suspected, the physician must look at the esophagus through a flexible gastroscope because inflammation (esophagitis) may not show on x-ray (see Chapter 22).

Esophageal motor studies are next in fashion, but as can be seen from the foregoing description, the results are often inconclusive; thus, provocative studies are advocated. The pain and the motility disturbances may be simultaneously reproduced by acid infusion, cholinergic stimulation by a drug (eg, edrophonium—a cholinesterase inhibitor; see Chapter 20), or by balloon distension within the esophagus. In the event of a positive result, the physician may be convinced, but such concordance is not the rule.

Longer studies, such as those employing 24-hour intraluminal esophageal acid and pressure recording systems, may help the physicians and patients to understand this condition better. By using a sensing device on a long tube that is placed in the esophagus above the LES, motility events are then recorded on tape, and the patient records episodes of pain by pressing a button. The patient wears this apparatus at home and goes about his or her customary routine. Association of pain with motility or reflux events are taken as positive evidence of esophageal chest pain. It should be remembered that only 10 percent to 20 percent of pain events are associated with motility abnormalities or acid reflux. Outside of research centers, this test is not yet practical.

TREATMENT

There is no satisfactory treatment of esophageal chest pain. A trial of antireflux measures may help those individuals whose pain seems to be triggered by gastric acid (Chapter 10). A nitroglycerin tablet under the tongue is helpful in some individuals for a while, whereas those who are anxious or depressed may benefit from tranquilizers or antidepressants.

Nifedipine, a drug used for coronary artery spasm, blocks calcium influx into the muscle cell and thereby inhibits contraction (see Chapter 20). Perhaps the drug might improve esophageal pain since it lowers LES pressure and decreases esophageal contractions in the nutcracker esophagus. However, nifedipine has proven no better than placebo in reducing chest pain frequency or severity. Again, these observations demonstrate the uncertain relationship of esophageal contractions to chest pain.

Bougienage consists of the passage of mercury-weighted dilators through the esophagus. A double-blind, crossover trial of therapeutic bougienage (large bougie) and placebo bougienage (small bougie) demonstrated that they improved patients equally. It is certainly a possibility that the close physician–patient interaction necessitated by bougienage may be more important therapy than the size of the bougie—a fundamental point that will be much emphasized in this book.

Germane to the above, the Bowman Gray group in their nifedipine trial presented evidence that noncardiac chest pain improves over 1 to 2 years. In another study over 22 months, they followed 119 patients of whom 63 had esophageal pain according to their criteria. All patients continued to have pain, but those 63 who were convinced that the esophagus was the cause were less disabled and required less physician care. A large part of a physician's business is reassurance.

SUMMARY

The irritable esophagus may be present in up to one third of patients with noncardiac chest pain, yet the mechanism is obscure. Association of abnormal esophageal pressure recordings with pain is the exception rather than the rule, and both are evidently influenced by stresses and particularly by the emotions. There is growing realization that the pain may be due at least partially to altered perception of esophageal events rather than to the events themselves. X-rays of the esophagus using barium, and/or endoscopy should be done to detect any structural disease. Since there is no treatment proven to be effective, motility studies are only justified for their placebo effect and for the reassurance that a positive study may engender in someone who is fearful of a bad heart. In the end, as with all manifestations of the irritable gut, time, good patient–physician interaction, consideration of contributing stressors, and maximum use of reassurance constitute the best medicine.

Heartburn

[A] sense of burning or smarting heat usually denominated heartburn.

Caleb Parry (1815)

Heartburn is a burning discomfort usually experienced behind the breastbone. Certain foods, anger, fear, reclining, or bending aggravate it, and the swallowing of food or an antacid may relieve it. This common symptom is familiar to most people and is easily understood, but its cause is far from simple. At least one third of the readers of this book will recognize this symptom in themselves.

EPIDEMIOLOGY

In our interviews of 301 apparently healthy Britons, Dr. Kenneth Heaton and I found that heartburn occurred in 33 percent of young, middle-aged, and elderly men and women. A survey of American hospital employees produced a similar result. This figure of 33 percent is so consistent that I am regularly able to demonstrate it among student and physician audiences by asking sufferers to raise their hands. Ten percent of our respondents had heartburn

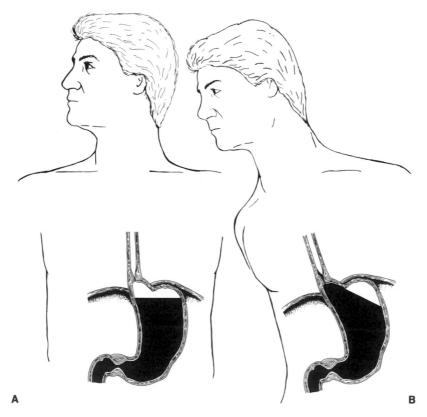

Figure 14. Effect of position on gastroesophageal reflux. (A) Upright position with gastric juice in the dependent part of the stomach. (B) Bending over. Gastric juice covers the cardia and may reflux through an incompetent LES. The hiatus hernia (shown here) may be irrelevant.

once a month. Daily heartburn occurs in 3 percent and 7 percent of Britons and Americans, respectively.

Hiatus hernia, which is a bulging of part of the stomach through the diaphragm into the chest (Figure 14), occurs in 30 percent of asymptomatic individuals. It is not surprising, therefore, that these two common conditions, heartburn and hiatus hernia,

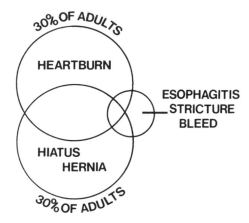

Figure 15. Venn diagram illustrating the relative prevalence and relationships of heartburn, hiatus hernia, and the severe complications of gastroesophageal reflux.

may occur together. But this fact has led to the fallacious view that
heartburn is *due* to a hiatus hernia, and some patients are accustomed to complain of their hiatus hernia rather than their heartburn. Clearly, heartburn occurs in the absence of a hiatus hernia,
and many people have a hernia with no heartburn. The relationship between these two entities and esophagitis (inflammation of
the esophagus) is shown in Figure 15 and is discussed further in
the next section.

In their East Africa mission, Burkitt and his colleagues (1973)
observed that natives rarely possessed a hiatus hernia, whereas
Americans of African descent have it as frequently as their white
compatriots. This finding led him to suggest that hernias result
from our Western-processed, fiber-deficient diet. For example, the
straining by a person to eject constipated, fiber-deficient stools can
generate 200 mm of mercury pressure within the abdomen, which
may by sufficient to push the stomach through the diaphragm.
However, we do not know the prevalence of heartburn in African
natives or the relationship of heartburn to straining or fiber ingestion.

GASTROESOPHAGEAL REFLUX DISEASE (GERD)

Mechanism

GERD refers to the consequences of the reflux of gastric or even duodenal contents from the stomach retrograde through the lower esophageal sphincter (LES) into the esophagus (Figure 14). Recordings from acid sensors (such as pH recording) in the lower esophagus indicate that reflux occurs in normal persons several times a day without producing symptoms. In many people, reflux causes heartburn and in a few it causes esophagitis. The principal barrier to reflux is the sphincter itself; however, the LES is not enough. This star of antireflux has a large supporting cast. Secondary peristalsis in the body of the esophagus acts as a housekeeper, promptly sweeping any refluxed stomach contents back to where they belong. Swallowed saliva, which is alkaline, may also help neutralize any refluxed acid. Brisk gastric antral motility may favor eflux rather than reflux of gastric contents. The hormone *gastrin*, produced by the antrum of the stomach to stimulate gastric secretion, also tightens the LES. Finally, the situation of the gastroesophageal junction below the diaphragm may be important (see Chapter 1). The sharp angle of Hiss between the esophagus and stomach, the pinchcock effect of the esophagus by the muscles of the diaphragm (see Figure 4), and the squeeze that is due to intra-abdominal pressure on the LES all help prevent reflux. In 1971, LES incompetence was declared unrelated to a hiatus hernia. This pronouncement gradually curtailed surgical repair of the hernia as a treatment for GERD. As in most things, however, the pendulum has swung back a little, and repair along with a sphincter-reenforcing operation seems a reasonable recourse in those severe cases of reflux esophagitis refractory to other measures.

Consequences of GERD

Reflux appears to occur harmlessly in normal people, but in some it has serious consequences. Reflux of gastric contents into the mouth risks aspiration into the lungs, and is an infrequent cause of asthma attacks or pneumonia. More commonly, acid and pepsin from the stomach may digest the squamous (flat) esophageal epithelium, which is not designed to contain acid. The resulting inflammation is called *esophagitis*. In severe cases of esophagitis, bleeding can cause acute blood loss or chronic anemia. Recurrent esophagitis may result in scarring and narrowing of the esophagus (stricture), which may impair swallowing (dysphagia). Chronic esophagitis may cause the flat squamous esophageal epithelium to become columnar (comprised of tall columnlike cells, such as are seen in the stomach or small gut). This condition is called *Barrett's esophagus*, and many researchers consider it to be precancerous. As discussed in Chapter 9, reflux may also induce esophageal motility abnormalities in patients with noncardiac chest pain.

The consequence of GERD that concerns us here is heartburn. Although esophagitis is commonly seen in gastroenterology clinics, it is not nearly as prevalent as is heartburn in the community. Heartburn and esophagitis are independent variables that have GERD in common. Thus heartburn and hiatus hernia, those very prevalent and largely independent phenomena, are seldom accompanied by esophagitis; yet esophagitis may occur without either (Figure 15). Because esophagitis is not a functional disorder, we will not consider it further. Rather, we will be concerned with those patients who have heartburn without endoscopic or histologic evidence of inflammation or structural change—a limit applicable to most individuals with mild or occasional heartburn.

What Causes Heartburn?

Some researchers might quarrel with the designation of heartburn as a functional disorder. "Is not GERD the culprit?" they might ask. "We know the cause." I do not think, however, that we do know the mechanism. Although GERD may be *sine qua non*, many refluxers do not have heartburn and even some with severe esophagitis have no symptoms. There does not appear to be an acid-induced motility disorder of the lower esophagus that coincides with the acid-induced pain. Irritation of nerves in the esophageal mucosa by refluxed acid might cause heartburn, but no such nerves have been found. The vagus nerve carries sensory impulses from the esophagus to the base of the brain, but we do not know how these impulses are generated. Doubtless, nerve endings in the esophageal muscle are important in coordinating motor activity, such as LES relaxation in response to a swallow. They could transmit a sensation of heartburn in response to altered muscle tone or altered sensitivity. In chronic reflux, some researchers report that processes called *papillae*, which indent the epithelium from below, come nearer the surface. Thus, nerve receptors (if they could be found) in the papilla might be more sensitive to acid. But other researchers report this same finding in normal people. Thus, until the link between events in the esophagus and consciousness is demonstrated, heartburn without esophagitis is a functional disorder.

FACTORS THAT CONTRIBUTE TO OR WORSEN HEARTBURN

In a person suffering from heartburn, aggravating features are generally those that encourage gastroesophageal reflux. Some, but not all, sufferers have decreased LES pressures. As discussed in Chapter 2, LES function is subject to a bewildering array of neural and humoral influences that interact with one another and with various foods, tobacco, alcohol, and emotion. Although permutations and combinations of these variables are beyond the scope of this discussion, it is important to stress that no single factor should be taken in isolation. Someday we may have a simple scheme of LES dysfunction and heartburn, but do not count on it being soon. Meanwhile, the principles of heartburn therapy center upon keeping gastric contents out of the esophagus.

Mechanical Factors

Delayed emptying of the stomach, such as one might see in an individual with a peptic ulcer or a scar at the pylorus, might encourage reflux. In most sufferers, however, no abnormal gastric motility is observed. But obesity can contribute to reflux by compressing the stomach. On the other hand, the heartburn of pregnancy occurs when the fetus is still in the pelvis and may be due to LES impairment by the hormone progesterone. Furthermore, straining at stool, exercise, or lifting can increase intra-abdominal pressure, which, in turn, may overcome pressure in the LES, especially if the LES is not below the diaphragm. If the sphincter is lax, gravity may overcome the gastroesophageal barrier when an individual bends or reclines. The degree of esophageal damage and perhaps the severity of heartburn are related to the frequency of reflux events, the volume and potency of the refluxed material (acid, bile salts), the efficiency of esophageal clearance by peristalsis, the resistance of the esophageal mucosa, and the volume of neutralizing saliva.

Dietary Factors

Even a modest gain in weight may induce heartburn. Protein meals increase LES tone, whereas fats relax the sphincter and retard gastric emptying. Alcohol, tobacco, and coffee (even decaffeinated) cause heartburn by reducing sphincter tone. Peppermint is a smooth muscle relaxant which, like chocolate, is often offered as an after-dinner digestive. The heartburn sufferer should beware of peppermint and chocolate since both relax the LES. Onions and garlic have similar effects. Because concentrated solutions of sugar or salt may irritate a sensitive esophagus, this factor, rather than their weak acid content, may explain why juices are poorly tolerated.

Drugs

Many heartburn sufferers along with their physicians are unaware that several drugs may exacerbate reflux and heartburn. Progesterone-containing oral contraceptives, aspirin (acetylsalicylic acid), other nonsteroidal analgesic drugs, theophylline, and such anticholinergic drugs as those used for Parkinson's disease may provoke or worsen heartburn (see Chapter 20). Many drugs used for such mental disorders as schizophrenia or depression have anticholinergic properties. Thus, the phenothiazine group of drugs and the tricyclic antidepressants may encourage reflux by decreasing esophageal peristalsis, reducing LES tone, and slowing gastric emptying. Drugs with β_1- and β_2-adrenergic activity, such as terbutaline, reduce esophageal peristalsis. Thus, the importance of drug review in the heartburn sufferer is obvious (Chapter 20).

Emotion

How tartly that gentleman looks!
I never can see him, but I am
Heartburned an hour after.

Much Ado about Nothing (2.1)

Certainly, Shakespeare recognized the effect of emotion on the esophagus. Anxiety or fear are aggravating factors to many. As with all syndromes of the irritable gut, a sufferer's psychological status is important in the manifestation of symptoms. Even the self-confident Beatrice in *Much Ado* experienced heartburn when she was distressed.

DIAGNOSIS

History

The burning nature of the retrosternal pain, its relief with antacids, its relation to bending, and its association with regurgitation all serve to identify heartburn in most sufferers. Some patients describe the discomfort as a "lump" in the chest; a small minority report a tight or gripping pain. Since the esophagus is served by nerves that also supply the heart, occasionally the pain may resemble heart pain (angina), radiating even to the neck or arm. As discussed in the previous chapter, such pain leads the patient to be seen by a cardiologist. To add to the confusion with angina, some individuals with heartburn report that it is worse with exercise or emotion and is relieved by rest. Although usually retrosternal, the discomfort of heartburn may be felt in the epigastrium (upper belly) and be mistaken for ulcer or nonulcer dyspepsia. Of course, more than one of these conditions may occur in the same person. Gallbladder pain is usually experienced in the right upper corner of the abdomen and penetrates through to the back. Although it may occasionally occur in the chest, the discrete, irregular, devastating attacks serve to distinguish it from heartburn. Pain from the chest wall was discussed in Chapter 9.

Many patients relate their symptoms to anxiety or to certain foods. It is the effect of bodily position, however, that most reliably pins down gastroesophageal reflux as the cause of retrosternal discomfort. After a large meal, the stomach contains acid and food, a condition that is ideal for discharge into the esophagus. Recumbency, especially after a meal, is frequently a precipitating factor. Thus, many sufferers report heartburn when they bend over to pick up something, tie their shoelaces, or scrub the floor. One may imagine the stomach being somewhat like a teapot, emptying through the esophageal spout—an action that may be given extra impetus by abdominal muscles which become tightened with effort (Figure 14).

Most people with infrequent heartburn do not consult a doctor for it, nor should they. A physician may be helpful when the symptom is worrying to the person or when it interferes with normal living. In a well-nourished person with a typical heartburn history, it is reasonable to try to relieve symptoms without further investigation. Since one third of the population has heartburn, it is not practical to perform endoscopy on everyone who complains of it.

Difficulty swallowing (dysphagia) is a worrying symptom to

the physician. Seldom, if ever, functional, it may signify severe inflammation, stricture, or cancer of the esophagus, and endoscopy should be done without delay. Gastrointestinal bleeding is also an indication for investigation. Bleeding caused by esophagitis is usually slow and may result in an iron-deficiency anemia. Rarely is blood passed or vomited. Atypical or intractable heartburn or accompanying weight loss, chest pain, or dysphagia also require further investigation.

Investigation

Generally, blood is taken for a hemoglobin estimation to ensure that a patient has not been bleeding. A barium x-ray examination of the esophagus, stomach, and duodenum is often ordered, especially if endoscopy is not readily available, because it helps to exclude structural lesions, such as strictures, tumors, and ulcers. Remember that unless a hernia is huge, its discovery is irrelevant. Further, barium examination will not identify esophagitis and may not distinguish ulcers and strictures from tumors. For this reason, endoscopy is the preferred examination (see Chapter 22).

In experienced hands, fiberoptic esophagoscopy is a safe and productive examination. Erosive esophagitis can easily be recognized, and, occasionally, incompetence of the LES may be observed. If a stricture is present, the appearance of the lesion and biopsy should exclude cancer. The presence of intraesophageal columnar epithelium (Barrett's esophagus) may also be observed. Finally, with this examination, the physician may exclude esophageal, gastric, or duodenal ulcers.

Sometimes, a physician cannot be sure whether or not chest discomfort in a patient is due to GERD. Such puzzling pains can, at times, be clarified through the use of the esophageal acid-perfusion test. In this test, a small tube is placed in the upper esophagus. Three solutions, isotonic saline, hydrochloric acid, and sodium bicarbonate (antacid), are slowly perfused in sequence. Saline should elicit no response; but acid may reproduce the patient's discomfort, which, in turn, is relieved by the antacid. A positive test is very good evidence that the patient's discomfort is due to gastroesophageal reflux.

Esophageal manometry (pressure recording) is of doubtful value in the routine investigation of heartburn (see Chapter 9). Not only can it produce chaotic information for the inexperienced manometrist, but it is also fraught with many technical difficulties about which the pundits disagree. Simple LES pressure recording will misclassify one half of individuals. Nevertheless, if an antireflux operation is contemplated, motility is required to point out any defect in acid-clearing peristalsis, such as in scleroderma, or to identify esophageal spasm. Such defects predict poor surgical results, since a reinforced LES may impair the ability to swallow.

As we described in Chapter 9, the 24-hour pH (acid) and motility recording of the lower esophagus makes it possible to correlate esophageal events with symptoms. However, more experience with this device is required before it can be recommended for general use. Some centers employ gastroesophageal scintiscanning techniques to demonstrate esophageal emptying and reflux. The examinee is instructed to drink orange juice containing gamma-emitting technetium 99 sulfur colloid. The juice's progress through the esophagus and stomach is then monitored by a gamma camera. As we have stressed in the previous section, the vast majority of heartburn sufferers do not need any of these tests.

MANAGEMENT

A sufferer may easily grasp the management of heartburn if he or she remembers how it occurs. Treatment is based upon reducing the contact of gastric acid, pepsin, and duodenal juice with the esophagus. No two patients are alike, and therapy must be individualized. There is no point in having a patient chew an antacid at a time when he or she is unlikely to have heartburn, or in removing an item from the sufferer's diet when it is clearly not the source of the discomfort.

Diet

Since a large meal will remain in the stomach for several hours, thereby increasing the opportunity for gastroesophageal reflux, sufferers should distribute their intake over 3 or 4 meals. Food likely to stimulate gastric acid secretion, such as alcohol and beef broth, should be avoided. Fatty foods can slow gastric emptying, thus prolonging the period of possible regurgitation, but a low-fat diet is both difficult and uninteresting. Drugs with anticholinergic effects, coffee, chocolate, onions, and alcohol should be withdrawn. During the acute phase, it also makes sense to avoid mechanical irritation by coarse, very hot, or very cold foods. Further, it is wise to resist such spices as hot chili or curry. Many physicians recommend that beverages be taken separately from the meals because dry food is less likely to reflux. Overweight sufferers should also see a dietitian for weight-losing advice. Although tobacco is not food, it may as well be proscribed in this section as anywhere else. Like alcohol, it stimulates gastric secretion and adversely affects the LES. In fact, smoking has nothing to recommend it except, perhaps, the taxes it generates to support research into its harmful effects.

Posture

Because gravity can help keep gastric contents out of the esophagus, the heartburn sufferer should adopt postures that maintain the esophagus higher than the stomach and that minimize external pressure on the stomach. For the sufferer of nocturnal heartburn, this implies elevation of the head of the bed on 6- to 8-inch blocks (Figure 16). Unfortunately, this elevation may inspire a protest from the sufferer's spouse who, not motivated by sleepless heartburn, may slide off the bed. Despite this "slide effect," elevation of the head of the bed is superior to other arrangements. Some heartburn sufferers experience relief by elevating their head with a pillow, but the resulting jackknife position may exert pressure on the stomach and nullify the benefit of gravity.

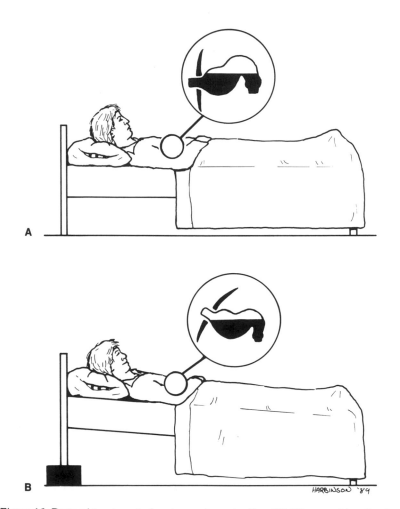

Figure 16. Postural treatment of gastroesophageal reflux. (A) When a subject lies flat in bed, gastric contents overlie the esophagogastric junction. If the lower esophageal sphincter is weak, reflux of gastric contents into the esophagus may occur. (B) Elevation of the head of the bed on an 8-inch block places the esophagus above the stomach. Gravity maintains gastric contents below the esophagus, thus avoiding reflux.

For those sufferers with waterbeds, another solution must be obtained.

Normally, gastroenterologists, like governments, have no place in the bedrooms of the nation. A recent report from Glasgow, Scotland, entitled *Reflux Dyspareunia*, forces an exception to that rule. It appears that 77 of 100 women surveyed in that city reported heartburn during sexual intercourse. Simple measures, such as weight reduction, avoiding stooping, and the use of the female superior position, resulted in improvement in 61 of the 77 victims. (Sorry, no illustration!)

The "teapot" effect of bending over may be avoided if the individual lifts from the knees, thus maintaining a vertical spine, a precaution recommended for patients with back pain that is due to vertebral disk disease. After a meal, bending and recumbency should be particularly avoided. Pressure on the abdomen, too, might be minimized by forgoing tight clothes, belts, and girdles.

Drug Therapy

As with other functional disorders, drug therapy for heartburn should be minimized. Such a common, usually hazardless symptom should not be treated with agents that might produce results far worse than the disease. However, heartburn is nearer the frontier between functional and organic disease than the other irritable gut syndromes. Further, we know that reflux of gastric acid into the esophagus may be complicated by esophagitis. It therefore makes sense to neutralize the acid in the esophagus with antacids. There are many newer, potent drugs that reduce acid secretion, or protect the esophageal mucosa, or prevent reflux, or ensure quick exit of any refluxed material. Usually, these drugs should be reserved for esophagitis.

Antacids

One method of mitigating the harmful effects of refluxed hydrochloric acid in the esophagus is to neutralize it in the stomach and esophagus with an antacid. Many heartburn sufferers discover relief on their own and chew Tums or Rolaids obtained from the pharmacist. Although the effect of alkalinization of gastric contents on LES function is in some scientific dispute, nevertheless, the sufferer should be aware that the peppermint that is frequently used to flavor the antacid is an LES relaxant. Scientific uncertainties aside, antacids do relieve heartburn. Tablets must be thoroughly chewed in order to maximize dispersal in the esophagus and stomach. Liquid antacids are preferable but less convenient.

How does the heartburn sufferer select from the bewildering array of preparations that glut pharmacists' shelves? It would help to be familiar with the four commonly used inorganic antacids: sodium bicarbonate, calcium carbonate, magnesium hydroxide, and aluminum hydroxide. Factors to be considered in the quest for a perfect antacid include its neutralizing power, expense, sodium content, effect on the bowels, and its effect on absorption or metabolism of drugs and minerals (Tables 9 and 10).

Bicarbonate. Sodium bicarbonate is not an ideal antacid because it is weakly effective and may produce, in large doses, systemic alkalosis. The sodium content makes it undesirable in some cardiac patients. Through its reaction with stomach acid, carbon dioxide gas production may generate a satisfying burp in some individuals but distress in others. Commonly known as baking soda, sodium bicarbonate is a cheap and effective home remedy and is the active ingredient in many patent seltzers. Its use should not be entirely discouraged, so long as it is used in moderation; that is, 1 to 2 teaspoons per day.

At fine European restaurants, a bottle of *l'eau minérale gaseuse* has a prominent place next to the local wine. These mineral waters contain up to 5 grams per liter of bicarbonate. Often their labels boast of their ability to regularize "l'activité hepatobilaire." More likely, they owe their popularity to their acid-neutralizing effects.

Calcium Carbonate. Calcium carbonate (Tums, Titralac) is the most powerful antacid in the test tube. It is cheap and has been used in the form of chalk powder or oyster shell for centuries. Many

Table 9

Characteristics of Some Liquid Antacids[a]

Product	Ingredients[b] (milligram/ 5 milliliters)	Acid-neutralizing capacity (milliequivalents/ 5 milliliters)	Sodium content (milligram/ 5 milliliters)	Calorie content (milligram/ 5 milliliters)	Average (1985) price to pharmacist per 100 milliliter ($ can)
High					
Mylanta-2 Extra Strength	$Al(OH)_3$ 650 $Mg(OH)_2$ 350 Simethicone 30	32.34	1.0	1.3	1.21
Amphojel 500	$Al(OH)_3$ 500 $Mg(OH)_2$ 500	31.92	2.5	2.4	1.18
Gelusil Extra Strength	$Al(OH)_3$ 650 $Mg(OH)_2$ 350	31.90	0.8	1.3	1.16
Intermediate-high					
Maalox TC	$Al(OH)_3$ 600 $Mg(OH)_2$ 300	27.06	1.0	3.0	1.13
Diovol Ex	$Al(OH)_3$ 600 $Mg(OH)_2$ 300	26.84	2.2	4.6	1.06
Intermediate					
Amphojel Plus	$Al(OH)_3$ 300 $Mg(OH)_2$ 300 Simethicone 25	20.40	6.0	2.4	0.77
Titralac	$CaCO_3$ 1000	19.71	11.0	1.2	1.06
Camalox	$Al(OH)_3$ 225 $Mg(OH)_2$ 200 $CaCO_3$ 250	18.24	1.0	1.0	1.19

Low

Product	Composition			
Phillips' Milk of Magnesia	Mg(OH)$_2$ 408	13.95	NA	Nil	0.59
Maalox	Al(OH)$_3$ 228 Mg(OH)$_2$ 200	13.50	0.9	0.2	0.89
Diovol	Al(OH)$_3$ 200 Mg(OH)$_2$ 200 Simethicone 25	13.38	2.9	2.6	0.84
Antacid Plus	Al(OH)$_3$ 200 Mg(OH)$_2$ 200 Simethicone 25	13.31	7.0	3.6	NA
Diovol (fruit flavored)	Al(OH)$_3$ 200 Mg(OH)$_2$ 200 Simethicone 25	13.20	9.2	2.6	0.84
Maalox Plus	Al(OH)$_3$ 228 Mg(OH)$_2$ 200 Simethicone 25	12.85	0.9	0.9	1.00
Univol	Al(OH)$_3$ 200 Mg(OH)$_2$ 200	12.75	10.6	2.3	0.73
Gelusil	Al(OH)$_3$ 200 Mg(OH)$_2$ 200	12.49	1.8	2.3	0.96
Mylanta	Al(OH)$_3$ 200 Mg(OH)$_2$ 200 Simethicone 20	12.42	5.0	2.8	0.95
DiGel	Al(OH)$_3$ 296.5 Mg(OH)$_2$ 87	11.72	9.4	1.8	0.90
Rioplus	Magaldrate 400 Simethicone 20	11.29	0.7	1.1	0.90
Riopan	Magaldrate 400	10.38	0.7	1.1	0.86
Amphojel	Al(OH)$_3$ 320	10.17	9.5	1.4	0.77

[a] Adapted from the *Canadian Medical Association Journal* (1985;132:523–527).
[b] Al = aluminum; Mg = magnesium; Ca = calcium.

Table 10
Characteristics of Some Tablet Antacids[a]

Product	Ingredients[b] (milligram per tablet)	Acid-neutralizing capacity (milliequivalent per tablet)	Sodium content (milligram per tablet)	Calorie content (milligram per tablet)	Average (1985) price to pharmacist for 10 tablets ($ can)
Maalox	$Al(OH)_3$ 400 $Mg(OH)_2$ 400	23.3	0.9	1.2	0.70
Amphojel	$Al(OH)_3$ 600	22.2	0.9	0.8	0.75
Gelusil-400	$Al(OH)_3$ 400 $Mg(OH)_2$ 400	19.9	1.8	3.8	0.58
Mylanta-2	$Al(OH)_3$ 400 $Mg(OH)_2$ 400 Simethicone 30	19.3	1.8	Nil	0.92
Camalox	$Al(OH)_3$ 225 $Mg(OH)_2$ 200 $CaCO_3$ 250	18.0	1.5	1.3	1.02
Amphojel Plus	$Al(OH)_3$ 300 $MgCO_3$ 300 $Mg(OH)_2$ 300 Simethicone 25	17.6	5.3	2.9	0.75
Univol	$Al(OH)_3$ 300 $MgCO_3$ 300 $Mg(OH)_2$ 100	12.5	7.1	1.0	0.58

Maalox Plus	Al(OH)$_3$ 200 Mg(OH)$_2$ 200 Simethicone 25	11.7	0.9	2.8	0.70
Gelusil	Al(OH)$_3$ 200 Mg(OH)$_2$ 200	11.4	0.5	2.8	0.87
Riopan	Magaldrate 400	11.2	0.7	1.1	0.63
Diovol	Al(OH)$_3$ 300 MgCO$_3$ 300 Mg(OH)$_2$ 100 Simethicone 25	11.2	6.4	2.5	0.66
Phillips' Milk of Magnesia	Mg(OH)$_2$ 310	10.8	NA	1.1	0.32
Tums	CaCO$_3$ 500	10.3	3.0	3.0	0.17
DiGel	Al(OH)$_3$ 282 MgCO$_3$ 282 Mg(OH)$_2$ 85 Dimethicone 25	9.9	11.7	0.4	0.85
Kolantyl	Al(OH)$_3$ 180 Mg(OH)$_2$ 170	8.6	1.9	4.3	0.75
Titralac	CaCO$_3$ 420	8.5	0.3	1.0	0.48
Rolaids	Dihydroxy aluminum sodium carbonate 334	8.4	48.0	5.9	0.18
Mylanta	Al(OH)$_3$ 200 Mg(OH)$_2$ 200 Simethicone 20	7.5	0.4	Nil	0.72

[a] Adapted from the *Canadian Medical Association Journal* (1985;132:523–527).
[b] Al = aluminum; Mg = magnesium; Ca = calcium.

physicians consider it potentially constipating. Further, calcium ions may be absorbed and result in hypercalcemia, particularly in patients with kidney failure. Nonetheless, calcium carbonate is often preferred over other antacids.

Magnesium Hydroxide. Magnesium hydroxide, or milk of magnesia, is a familiar laxative and is probably the safest effective antacid. Some magnesium is absorbed so that hypermagnesemia is a hazard in kidney failure. For most patients, however, the greatest disadvantage of magnesium is its laxative effect. For this reason, it is commonly combined with aluminum hydroxide, which reduces the neutralizing capacity of the combination and doubles the price (see below). Prolonged use of magnesium hydroxide impairs phosphorus absorption and may cause hypercalcemia and loss of bone calcium and phosphorus. Finally, magnesium hydroxide may alter the absorption of some other drugs.

Aluminum Hydroxide. Hydrated aluminum hydroxide, given in the form of a gel, is a slow-acting antacid. Aluminum toxicity has received some attention lately as a possible cause of Alzheimer's disease, but no connection has been proven. Aluminum forms an insoluble compound with dietary phosphate, and kidney specialists take advantage of this characteristic to prevent the high blood phosphate of kidney failure. Aluminum hydroxide also interferes with the absorption of drugs, such as digoxin, tetracycline, and atropine. This antacid causes constipation particularly in the elderly. Of the commonly used antacids it is the least effective neutralizer.

There are no data available to support the usefulness of aluminum hydroxide alone in the treatment of heartburn. However, this antacid does bind bile acids. If bile acids are important in the genesis of heartburn as, for example, after gastric surgery, then aluminum hydroxide would seem to be the antacid of choice.

Combination Antacids. Because no single antacid ingredient is perfect, there are many combinations. Most consist of magnesium hydroxide combined with aluminum or calcium in order to balance the laxative and constipating effects and minimize other undesirable reactions. Combinations are expensive, and antacid objectives could be achieved more economically by suggesting that the patient alternate milk of magnesia with calcium carbonate tablets or aluminum hydroxide gel. The salt content of antacids varies, but low-sodium values sometimes accompany low potency (see Tables 9 and 10).

Neutralizing power varies among the common antacid preparations. For example, 5 milliliters (1 teaspoonful) of Mylanta neutralizes 32.34 millicquivalents of hydrochloric acid. Maalox, which contains magnesium and aluminum hydroxide, is less potent. Amphojel, containing aluminum hydroxide, and Gelusil, containing magnesium trisilicate, have even less neutralizing capacity. Some manufacturers increase potency by increasing the concentration of the ingredients. Such maneuvers are based more on marketing than on science. A rule of thumb is to choose a standard, inexpensive magnesium–aluminum preparation with no frills.

Local anesthetics, such as oxethazaine, given orally are believed to reduce acid secretion by blocking gastrin release from the gastric mucosa. Added to antacids, oxethazaine relieves ulcer pain faster than antacid alone, but the ingredient is seldom necessary.

An imaginative preparation consisting of antacid plus sodium alginate (Gaviscon) has been developed for the treatment of heartburn. The alginate floats, as a neutral raft of algae on a sea of gastric juice, and "corks" the cardia. If reflux does occur, it is of alginate and antacid, not acid.

Antacid Administration. Fifteen milliliters of antacid (one tablespoonful) may be taken for symptoms in those sufferers with irregular and occasional heartburn. For those individuals with predictable distress, it makes sense to take the antacid just before heartburn is expected, which is usually after meals, at bedtime, after alcohol consumption, or with exertion. Tablets are more convenient and cheaper than liquid antacids, but less easily dispersed. For example, the busy executive should be advised to keep tablets in a pocket and liquid antacid at the bedside, office desk, or with a lover.

As with the treatment of peptic ulcer, the timing of antacid administration is critical for its maximum effectiveness. If it is given 1 hour after a meal, some antacid will remain in the stomach for 2 to 3 hours. Thus, it is logical to assume that the risk of reflux and heartburn is greatest during the period of maximum stomach acid content, which often occurs about 1 hour after meals while the stomach is emptying, and at night. Therefore, for the maximum length of effect, the antacid should be given after meals and before the onset of discomfort so as to anticipate acid–pepsin activity. However, not all heartburn sufferers exhibit this typical pattern, so antacid administration must be tailored to the individual.

H_2 Antagonists

Cimetidine (Tagamet), the first commercial H_2 antagonist, represents one of the most remarkable advances in gastrointestinal drug therapy. Its discoverer, Sir James Black, received the 1988 Nobel Prize for medicine. Histamine acts to stimulate gastric acid and pepsin secretion but has numerous systemic effects as well, including flushing, rapid pulse, and low blood pressure. Standard antihistamines used for allergies, such as chlorpheniramine, block these untoward effects. In the histamine test of gastric acid production, histamine and antihistamines are given together to elicit a maximum gastric acid response to histamine without the systemic effects (Figure 17). These antihistamines are said to block the H_1 receptor. On the other hand, cimetidine, ranitidine, and the other H_2 antagonists block only the effect of histamine on stomach H_2 receptors.

One 600-milligram tablet of cimetidine twice daily or 150 milligrams of ranitidine (Zantac) twice daily are prompt, effective medications for the treatment of severe heartburn. They heal most esophagitis, but there is disagreement whether this healing benefits the fundamental motor abnormalities in the LES and lower esophagus. Relapses can occur, so some physicians prescribe a nocturnal dose as maintenance therapy.

However, the physician should ask whether it is sensible to

HISTAMINE

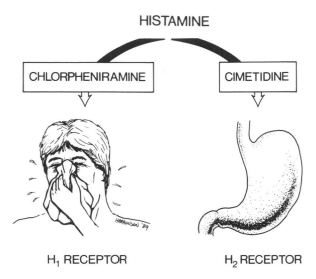

Figure 17. Histamine receptors. Standard antihistamines (eg, chlorpheniramine) block the effect of histamine on the H_1 receptors as exemplified by those in the nasal mucosa, where histamine mediates the allergic reaction in hay fever. They have no effect on the stomach. Cimetidine blocks only the H_2 receptors, which are mainly found on the acid-producing (parietal) cells in the gastric mucosa.

use a potent, costly, systemic drug for the average case of heartburn, especially when one third of the population are sufferers and are likely to have it for long periods of their lives. No drug can be certified safe, even though the H_2 blockers are considered relatively safe. Even an accidental ingestion of ten times the weekly dose of cimetidine had no apparent effect. Nonetheless, as clinical experience with cimetidine has accumulated, some undesirable effects have become apparent, including lactation in women, impotence and breast development in men, and mental confusion in the elderly. Through effects on liver blood flow and the activity of a liver enzyme (cytochrome p 450), the metabolism of certain drugs can become impaired. Especially in the elderly, such altered drug handling may be critical, as in the use of theophylline (Theo-Dur) in asthma, or warfarin (Coumadin) for the prevention of blood clots.

These unusual side effects are so far unreported with ranitidine or famotidine (Pepcid), but experience with these drugs is far less. This is a very competitive field, where 1 percent of the market represents millions of dollars of profit for pharmaceutical houses. As citizens, doctors, and patients, we should critically examine the use of these drugs, or, indeed, the need for new ones in a benign condition that affects one third of the people. Is it not frivolous to employ such expensive drugs with unknown long-term effects in the management of simple heartburn, in which diet, weight loss, antacids, and postural adjustments are usually satisfactory? Such pharmacotherapeutic promiscuity may induce changes we cannot now envision. Initial success with H_2 blockers may seduce the sufferer to long-term use, because pretreatment conditions favoring acid reflux can be expected to recur once the drug is withdrawn.

Sucralfate

The major appeal of sucralfate (Sulcrate) is that it is not absorbed from the gut and has no known systemic effects. It is constipating and may bind to other drugs thus impairing their absorption. Sucralfate was developed in the Orient to heal peptic ulcers. Evidently, it binds with injured or dead tissue in the base of an ulcer thus preventing the damaging effects of gastric juice. There are reported antipepsin and prostaglandin-promoting effects as well, leading proponents to apply a much-abused term *cytoprotection* (cell protection).

Sucralfate suspension has been found to be a useful alternative to H_2 blockers in the treatment of esophagitis, but it is costly overkill in the case of simple heartburn when no tissue damage can be demonstrated. The large, awkward tablets are hard to swallow and may not coat the esophagus. A liquid suspension is not yet available in North America.

Gastrokinetic Agents

Metoclopramide (Maxeran) stimulates gastric antral contraction, speeds gastric emptying, and appears to raise LES pressure. It may exert these effects through the release of acetylcholine from cholinergic nerve endings (see Chapter 20). These attributes are desirable in GERD. Some, but not all, studies support its use along with an H_2 blocker in the treatment of severe esophagitis. The usual dose is 10 milligrams three times a day before meals, but it should be adjusted to suit the symptoms. The larger dose necessary to raise LES pressure increases its untoward effects. Occasionally, drowsiness, apprehension, and palpitations occur with this drug. Stimulation of release of the pituitary hormone prolactin may cause lactation in women and gynecomastia (breast development) in men. Metoclopramide antagonizes anticholinergics and therefore should not be administered with psychoactive agents, such as the tricyclic antidepressants (see Chapter 20). Further, the hurried gastric emptying promoted by the drug may alter the absorption pattern of other drugs. Huge doses taken in a suicide attempt have not caused serious illness, but metoclopramide's big disadvantage is its occasional neurologic side effects. It may cause a tremor similar to that seen with Parkinson's disease, or other abnormal movements, some of them irreversible. These risks plus the cost of the drug should make the physician hesitate to use it in the treatment of simple heartburn.

In Canada and in Europe, domperidone (Motilium) has largely supplanted metoclopramide. It exerts its gastrokinetic (stomach-stimulating) effect through its ability to antagonize dopamine. Dopamine is a neurotransmitter, which, like acetylcholine, is important in nerve transmission in the upper gastrointestinal tract (see Chapter 20). Because the drug does not pass into the brain, its neurologic effects are not prominent. Less well studied than metoclopramide, domperidone may be helpful in severe esophagitis.

Cisapride is a new gastrokinetic drug that apparently acts on the myenteric nerves by a nonacetylcholine, nondopamine mechanism. The drug appears to stimulate the entire gut, but its interest here is that it improves esophageal and gastric motility. Although the drug is still in the developmental stage, small studies show that it can offer improvement in esophagitis. Diarrhea and borborygmi (bowel noises) are the only side effects reported so far.

Some studies convincingly show that the cholinergic agent bethanechol (Urecholine) relieves some patients with severe heartburn. This drug stimulates saliva production and increases LES pressure. But should the physician recommend use of a drug with widespread effects for such a localized area of dysfunction? Certainly, it has no place in the treatment of simple heartburn.

Other Drugs

Omeprazole is a new drug that shuts off gastric secretion. Its disadvantage is its great potency and thus its use in simple heartburn treatment is overkill. The anacid stomach may allow overgrowth of bacteria, which might produce serious side effects. Theoretically, cancer might result from bacterial products called *nitrosamines*.

Pirenzepine (Gastrozepin) is an anticholinergic drug that inhibits gastric secretion with minimal anticholinergic effect elsewhere. Nonetheless, any anticholinergic effect makes it a less favorable drug in the treatment of heartburn. Prostaglandins (Misoprostol), which are said to have protective effects on the gastric mucosa, have not been found to be useful in the esophagus.

Surgery

In severe, intractable esophagitis, especially if complicated by stricture or bleeding, it is necessary to turn to the surgeon for help. Some studies, most without controls, have demonstrated the effectiveness of various hiatus hernia repairs in relieving heartburn, even though the recurrence rate may be 30 percent to 50 percent in 2 years. Most techniques aim to secure a subdiaphragmatic location for the LES, where its antireflux activity is thought to be optimal. Modern surgery includes plastic repair of the gastroesophageal junction in which a stomach wraparound supports the LES. Once one of the most commonly performed operations, hiatus hernia repair is now seldom done.

In functional heartburn caused by reflux but without esophagitis, surgery should be considered only with caution and collective opinion. Postoperative mortality and morbidity are not negligible. Although heartburn can be very distressful in the absence of esophagitis, there is no imminently dangerous complication, and the distress may not be due solely to reflux. Patients whose heartburn is associated with psychiatric problems may achieve only transient benefit. Flatulent dyspeptics, unable to belch after most modern repairs, can be numbered among a surgeon's most ungrateful patients.

Frequently, gallstones and hiatus hernia coexist. It has been suggested that at cholecystectomy the opportunity should not be lost to repair a hernia. This proposal ignores the principles enunciated above and, in particular, focuses attention on the hernia and not the reflux. Surely, the hiatus hernia found at cholecystectomy is the same as any other hiatus hernia. Surgical repair is justified only with intractable esophagitis.

SUMMARY

Heartburn is due to reflux of gastric contents into the gullet. Such reflux occurs because of a functional disturbance of the lower esophagus; that is, inadequate LES pressure and inefficient acid-clearing peristalsis. Usually, heartburn is identified by its retrosternal burning quality, its occurrence after meals, its relief with antacids, its exacerbation with bending or lying, and accompanying occasional rumination. Because at least one third of the adult population experiences heartburn, it should be treated, in the first instance, by small portions of a high-fiber, low-fat diet, omitting alcohol, cigarettes, and hot or spicy foods. The obese must lose weight. Items that sufferers find irritating or that have been found to lessen LES pressure should be omitted as necessary, and it is important for them to understand how reflux occurs. The sufferer should be instructed in the use of antacids, alginate, posture, and elevation of the head of the bed at night in order to minimize contact of acid gastric contents with the esophageal mucosa. Correct management of other functional disturbances, particularly dyspepsia, belching, and constipation, may have a salutary effect on heartburn. H_2 blockers and gastrokinetic agents should be reserved only for severe cases of heartburn or for esophagitis.

Intractable heartburn, dysphagia, or bleeding demands investigation. Esophageal acid perfusion and barium meal are helpful, but only esophagoscopy can establish the presence or absence of esophagitis. Surgery for heartburn without esophagitis or other complication is unwise.

CHAPTER ELEVEN

Nonulcer Dyspepsia

How are we to explain this . . . disease that is not; this wealth of balsams for sufferings which cannot be named? Is there no distress to lull, no pain to lenify?

T. C. Allbutt (1884)

Dyspepsia defies accurate definition and yet has been part of our language for centuries. It is a syndrome often related to eating that includes epigastric pain, discomfort, bloating, and fullness. The epigastrium is the area below the breastbone often referred to as "the pit of the stomach." Many individuals with dyspepsia may complain of gas, nausea, vomiting, and heartburn, and some may even choose to call their symptoms "indigestion." Athough dyspepsia has many qualifying terms, such as "acid," "nervous," "functional," and "essential," they tell us little about the patient's complaint or its cause. *Ovarian, gallbladder,* and *appendiceal* dyspepsia are meaningless terms. The only consistent features of dyspepsia are its location in the epigastrium and its chronicity, periodicity, and relationship to eating, which leads the doctor to suspect a peptic ulcer. *Nonulcer dyspepsia* (NUD) then is a functional gastrointestinal disorder featured by chronic, recurrent, often

135

Table 11

Studies of Dyspeptic Patients without Abnormalities of the Upper
Gastrointestinal Tract[a]

Investigators	Year of report	Number of patients	Percentage with no lesion
Jones	1945	8,985	47
Friedman	1948	138	67
Williams	1957	775	60
Krag	1965	430	30
Edwards	1968	424	52
Davis	1968	1,663	47
Bonnevie	1971	114	26
Barnes	1974	56	40
Mollmann	1975	197	55
Oddsson	1977	188	47/38[b]
Horrocks	1978	360	14
Beavis	1978	110	33
Gear	1980	346	47
Priebe	1982	88	42
Mean			46[c]

[a] Adapted from the *Canadian Medical Association Journal* (1984;130:565–569).
[b] The higher figure was obtained after roentgenography, the lower one after endoscopy.
[c] The studies reported since 1975 are endoscopy controlled and the mean is 34 percent.

meal-related, epigastric discomfort that is initially suspected to be due to a peptic ulcer but subsequently found not to be.

EPIDEMIOLOGY

In Chapter 5 we saw that dyspepsia may occur in 5 percent to 10 percent of the population. Since World War II, there have been nearly 20 reports of patients presenting to clinics complaining of dyspepsia that is thought to represent peptic ulcer disease. Data from 14 representative reports are summarized in Table 11. Over the last 40 years, the proportion of dyspeptic patients in whom no ulcer was found has been between 30 percent and 55 percent. The overall proportion is 46 percent, whereas that from the studies reported since 1975 is 34 percent. This difference probably reflects the advent of fiberoptic gastroscopes that permit direct inspection of the stomach and duodenum, but could also reflect inherent differences in the study groups. For example, the first two studies were of wartime servicemen, the majority of whom had no ulcer. Could it be that hospitals were more attractive than foxholes? These reports leave no doubt that many cases of dyspepsia have no known organic explanation.

ULCER VERSUS NONULCER DYSPEPSIA

Some researchers suggest that dyspepsia is a syndrome of peptic ulcer symptoms that may occur with or without a hole (ulcer) in the mucosa of the stomach; that is, peptic ulcer disease is a continuum with nonulcer dyspepsia at one end of the spectrum and ulcer at the other. It seems more likely that we are dealing with two distinct entities: ulcer and nonulcer dyspepsia. *Peptic ulcer* is known to be a chronic recurring condition. Usually, the occurrence and recurrence of the ulcer is accompanied by recurrent dyspeptic symptoms. As a group, ulcer patients tend to have blood type O, a family history of ulcers, and stomachs that produce more acid than normal. Occasionally, ulcers bleed, obstruct the pylorus causing vomiting, or perforate precipitating an acute surgical emergency. Although these complications are serious and require active medical treatment with or without surgery, they are exceptional.

Nonulcer dyspepsia is also chronic and recurrent. Table 12 illustrates that many or most dyspeptic patients have the symptoms many years later. The development of an ulcer in this group of patients may be no more likely than in the normal population. Also, nonulcer dyspepsia is not associated with any blood type or increased stomach acid production. Furthermore, since no ulcer is present, it cannot bleed, obstruct, or perforate. Thus, ulcer and nonulcer dyspepsia are two distinct conditions posing distinct management problems.

Table 12
Studies of Patients with Unexplained Dyspepsia Who Developed
a Peptic Ulcer

Investigators	Year of report	Number of patients	Number of years of follow-up	Percentage still dyspeptic	Percentage who developed a peptic ulcer
Brummer	1959	102	5–6	66	12
Gregory	1972	102	6	24	3
Talley	1987	110	2	70	3

CAUSE OF NONULCER DYSPEPSIA

We do not know what causes the symptoms of dyspepsia. In the case of ulcer, symptoms are assumed to be due to a break in the integrity of the stomach or duodenal mucosa, thus exposing the underlying tissues to acid and pepsin. This condition might irritate sensory nerves or release chemical mediators that generate the sensation of pain. However, this thesis is weakened by the failure of direct infusion of acid into the ulcer to reproduce the patient's dyspepsia. In the case of nonulcer dyspepsia, no cohesive theory explains the discomfort or pain. There is no break in mucosal integrity and no exposure of underlying tissues.

A Motility Problem?

It is possible that the symptoms of nonulcer dyspepsia are due to abnormal motility of the upper gastrointestinal tract, analogous to the dysfunction of the lower gut that is believed to be responsible for the irritable bowel syndrome. Reflux of gastric contents through the pylorus into the stomach may or may not cause gastritis or gastric ulcer, but no one has satisfactorily shown an association between this reflux and symptoms. Moreover, one study suggests that duodenogastric reflux is a normal event, no more likely in gastric ulcer or nonulcer dyspepsia than in asymptomatic individuals.

Dyspepsia in patients with diabetes is sometimes attributed to delayed gastric emptying. Enteric nerve damage resulting from the diabetes leads to gastric paralysis that may be improved by certain gastrokinetic drugs that stimulate stomach activity. Some nonulcer dyspepsia patients may have a similar delay in gastric emptying but most do not, and symptoms are not clearly associated with this phenomenon.

Antral *tachygastria* occurs in some patients with postprandial upper gastrointestinal distress. It consists of an increased frequency of antral electrical slow waves (6 to 10 per minute compared with 3 to 4 per minute normally) and has been treated with drugs or surgery. The importance of this gastric dysrhythmia in dyspepsia awaits further study. Most dyspeptic patients are not as ill as those reported to have antal tachygastria and do not have an abnormal myoelectric pattern. As with other functional complaints, it remains uncertain whether dyspepsia is a normal perception of abnormal gastric physiology, or an abnormal perception of normal physiology.

An Infection?

An organism called *Helicobacter pylori* frequently is found in the mucosa of the gastric antrum. It appears to occur in 20 percent of people and its frequency increases with age. In South America, the prevalence of the organism in people is even greater. Evidence is accumulating that this organism causes or is permitted by inflammation of the gastric antrum (gastritis). The organism may be eradicated temporarily and the gastritis improved by compounds containing bismuth or the antibiotic erythromycin. Gastritis, however, is usually unaccompanied by dyspepsia and vice versa. One of the most hotly contested controversies in medicine today centers around the relationship between *Helicobacter pylori* and dyspepsia.

An organism that is so commonly found in normal people is

bound to be found in many dyspeptics. To date studies have not clearly implicated infection to dyspepsia. Although bismuth and antibiotics may improve the gastritis, the physician should not expect them to have anything beyond a placebo response in dyspepsia (see the section on treatment below).

A Gas Problem?

The belching, gaseous distension, and borborygmi (noisy bowels) that may accompany postprandial discomfort have led to the term *flatulent dyspepsia*. However, these symptoms may accompany a peptic ulcer or the irritable bowel syndrome or may occur by themselves (see Chapter 12). Most gas in the stomach originates from swallowed air.

A Diet Problem?

Dyspepsia is more often the effect of over eating and over drinking than of any other cause.

Beaumont (1833)

Dyspeptics often attribute their symptoms to their diets, yet dietary control is frustratingly elusive. Certainly, when an individual experiences dyspepsia repeatedly after consuming a certain food, it should be eliminated from the diet. However, the physician must discourage severely restricted diets that may impair nutrition. Dyspepsia is often attributed to fatty foods and fatty acids that delay gastric emptying. During digestion, triglycerides release carbon dioxide and fat releases cholecystokinin (CCK), a hormone that stimulates motility at various levels of the gut. Finally, we know that some patients with the irritable bowel syndrome have measurable late colonic contractions after the administration of fat. These phenomena may account for the epigastric distress that dyspeptic patients attribute to ingested fat.

A Drug Problem?

Nonsteroidal anti-inflammatory agents, especially acetylsalicylic acid (aspirin), cause dyspepsia, peptic ulcer, and gastritis. But other drugs, such as opiates, iron preparations, and digitalis, may also cause dyspepsia through unknown mechanisms. Alcohol and tobacco, important in the pathogenesis of peptic ulcer, may cause nonulcer dyspepsia as well, but beyond common experience, there is little evidence bearing on this supposition (see Chapter 20).

An Emotional Problem?

Deep sorrow occasionally produces dyspepsia.

Caleb Perry (1815)

Although scientific data are scarce, it is generally accepted that emotion is important in the genesis of dyspepsia. In Chapter 7, we saw that an army surgeon took advantage of the opportunity to study gastric phenomena in a patient who had a gunshot wound through the abdominal wall that exposed the stomach to view. When the patient experienced fear, anger, or illness, his stomach became pale and the secretion of gastric juice fell. More recent observations suggest different but no less striking gastric responses to strong emotion. We need to understand better how such physiologic changes cause symptoms, and how they might be controlled.

As in the case of the irritable bowel, the onset of nonulcer dyspepsia may be preceded by a threatening life-event. In all functional disorders, the emotional state of a person with dyspepsia must be considered, because the symptom itself may not be as important as the manner in which the sufferer reacts to it.

Dyspepsia is the ruin of most things: empires, expeditions and everything else.

Thomas De Quincey (1923)

NAUSEA AND VOMITING

Dyspepsia and other functional irritable gut syndromes may be accompanied by nausea and vomiting. In patients with functional abdominal pain, nausea is common. Vomiting may occur in those patients with anorexia nervosa and bulimia, topics which will not be discussed further.

Vomiting is essential for survival. Poisons or irritants are often ejected by a young animal which then learns to avoid the offending substance. Humans, too, may become nauseated or even vomit if a sight or smell reminds them of a similar experience in their youth. This reaction may come to express disgust for a person, place, or thing, as is seen, for example, in such expressions as "You make me sick," and "It's enough to make me throw up." It is probable that repeated, unprovoked vomiting without systemic or other upper gastrointestinal disease is due to an emotional disturbance. Many individuals experience nausea or even vomiting before an athletic event or public performance, and brides are said to be particularly susceptible to this infirmity.

Vomiting can also be learned. Conditioning is exemplified by the sailor who vomits when he steps on a ship at dockside. What started in the sailor as an inner-ear response to motion becomes a learned response to a neutral factor, the ship.

Vomiting must be distinguished from regurgitation. Some people regurgitate food into the mouth, chew it with relish as a cow chews her cud, and then cheerfully swallow it again. This quaint habit is termed *merycism* or *rumination*. It is an uncommon private pleasure and seldom a clinical complaint unless objected to by another person who is forced to view the procedure. In one family, a man, his son, and his grandson all ruminated, yet they managed to keep it a secret from each other. Hadji Ali from Cairo, Egypt, turned the habit of rumination to advantage by offering public performances. He could swallow 30 hazelnuts and an almond and then return any number of them at the audience's command. In another spectacular act, he swallowed kerosene and water. When regurgitated over a candle, the kerosene was ignited by the flame, and then the blaze was extinguished by the water. A fellow gastric gymnast from Germany specialized in alternately regurgitating live frogs and goldfish. Less theatrical regurgitation may occur if the upper as well as the lower esophageal sphincter is incompetent in patients with gastroesophageal reflux disease. Regurgitation of food can mimic vomiting in patients with esophageal obstruction. Medications, such as digitalis and narcotics; cerebral, cardiac, and metabolic diseases; and specific afflictions of the gastrointestinal tract can also cause vomiting. Projectile vomiting is a characteristic of pyloric obstruction, and the return of food that was eaten 6 hours before suggests a disorder of gastric emptying.

The appearance of clear fluid in the mouth is called *water brash*. It is due to reflex salivation and may accompany vomiting or other abdominal discomfort.

DIAGNOSIS

History

The physician may reach a diagnosis of dyspepsia (ulcer or nonulcer) only from the sufferer's description. Dyspepsia is a persistent or recurrent epigastric discomfort or pain often initiated or relieved by eating, which may lead a physician to suspect a peptic ulcer. Since pain or discomfort are very personal experiences, those sufferers with dyspepsia may choose different words to describe the nature of the pain. Such adjectives as "gnawing," "burning," "aching," and "boring" are often used but do not discriminate dyspepsia from other disorders, or an ulcer from a nonulcer. "Fullness" and "bloating" accompany several of the functional gut symptoms and may be more likely in nonulcer than in ulcer dyspepsia.

The timing of the pain is of more value than its description. It is often experienced intermittently over many years. Dyspepsia may also be meal-related. Typically, sufferers are uncomfortable after meals, but occasionally food brings relief. It is probable that most people experience dyspepsia sometime in their lives, perhaps after a dietary or alcoholic indiscretion.

Several researchers have attempted to identify those features of dyspepsia that would suggest a peptic ulcer. Some think ulcer pain is more severe, but one cannot measure severity. Nocturnal pain relieved by antacids, a family history of peptic ulcer disease, blood group O, or spring and fall exacerbations of the pain all tilt the diagnosis toward peptic ulcer. Of course, a history of ulcer complications, such as bleeding, vomiting, or perforation requiring surgery, makes the diagnosis easy. Otherwise, there is no reliable means with which the physician may distinguish ulcer from non-ulcer dyspepsia.

In contrast, it is possible to distinguish dyspepsia from other common causes of epigastric pain and discomfort. In the previous chapter, we noted that heartburn might be experienced in the epigastrium. It is well to remember that heartburn is due to the reflux of gastric contents into the esophagus and that it worsens with bending or lying, especially after a meal. The irritable bowel and constipation may also cause epigastric discomfort, and here the pain can be related to bowel action. Generally, the discomfort is improved or occasionally worsened with defecation, and the frequency and consistency of the stool may alter as the pain comes and goes (see Chapter 13).

In the past, some surgeons believed that dyspepsia might be caused by gallstones. Up to 20 percent of people have gallstones and many have no symptoms. Stones are more common in women, and the prevalence increases with age. Certain populations, such as the Pima Indians in the Western United States, are particularly liable to have gallstones. It is not surprising, therefore, that many individuals have both gallstones and dyspepsia. However, according to many studies, dyspepsia and "flatulence" are no more common in those who have gallstones than in those who do not. Most gallstones cause no trouble; however, when they obstruct the bile ducts, they may cause an attack of excruciating pain below the right rib cage, which is felt in the back and often requires narcotics for relief. Occasionally, jaundice or infection may intervene. Because gallstone attacks are unpredictable and usually occur weeks apart, they clearly are not dyspepsia.

If epigastric pain of recent onset is severe, persistent, and debilitating, particularly in an elderly person who shows such signs of failing health as weight loss, bleeding or vomiting, the physician must consider stomach or pancreatic cancer. Among dyspeptic patients, the risk of either is very small. Even though heart pain (angina) is rarely experienced in the epigastrium, it is easily recognized by its relationship to exercise and relief with rest. In patients with severe heart disease, rarely will abdominal pain result from insufficient blood supply to the intestine after meals. Several chronic epigastric pains that are not easily explained will be discussed in Chapter 14.

Physical Examination

There are no physical signs of dyspepsia. When a physician presses on a dyspeptic person's abdomen, it might be expected that if an ulcer were present he would elicit pain (tenderness); but this is not necessarily the case. Such tenderness is just as likely in ulcer or in nonulcer dyspepsia. Nevertheless, it is important that the physician examine the dyspeptic, because there may be signs of more serious disease present, such as an abdominal mass (lump) or heart disease.

Investigation

The diagnosis of gastralgia is, in certain stages, impossible.

Allbutt (1884)

The approach to the dyspeptic patient is still controversial, with the debate centering on cost versus benefits. Briefly stated, there is disagreement in the medical profession whether a complaint of dyspepsia should prompt a gastroscopy (Chapter 22) or a trial with powerful antiulcer medication. Like Allbutt 100 years ago, without endoscopy we cannot be sure whether or not an individual dyspeptic has an ulcer.

All researchers would agree that mild or occasional dyspepsia, especially in a young person, will usually respond to the recommendation of better eating habits and the symptomatic use of harmless antacids, such as Tums or Maalox. Further, the patient must withdraw such offending agents as alcohol, tobacco, and drugs, especially aspirin and antirheumatic agents. If these suggestions fail and the physician considers the use of powerful, systemic, costly, antiulcer drugs, he must also ask whether there is need to know if an ulcer is there or not.

The complication rate for gastroscopy is near zero, so risk is not a consideration, but cost is. Since in the United States endoscopy may cost up to $900, the American College of Physicians recommends that the proper course is a 6- to 8-week trial of therapy with an antiulcer drug such as ranitidine. If symptoms persist or recur, and if there are complications or a systemic illness, then endoscopy should be employed. To support their view, the college points out that many dyspeptics have no ulcer, the likelihood of cancer is remote, and both ulcer and nonulcer dyspepsia may improve with therapy.

There is a contrary view that may be more viable in jurisdictions in which universal Medicare is available or in which the cost of endoscopy is less. Both ulcer and nonulcer dyspepsia are chronic, recurring conditions and in both, an improvement in symptoms occurs with placebo in up to 50 percent of persons (see Chapter 21). Thus, no conclusions can be drawn from a successful or unsuccessful trial of therapy, and when the symptoms inevitably recur, the test will be required anyway. Further, since ulcer dyspepsia responds to medication better than placebo, whereas nonulcer dyspepsia does not, the most effective therapeutic tool in the latter case is reassurance made possible by a positive diagnosis. Finally, no drug is harmless and the cost of antiulcer drugs is not small. At $50 a month when administered for a chronic condition, drug costs may soon overtake the cost of a single, initial endoscopy. Many studies attest to the inappropriate long-term use of these drugs, especially in the elderly, where medication errors and interactions are common.

Although neither of the above approaches is wrong, the physician needs to use common sense and consider local circumstances. For example, although endoscopy is most accurate, a carefully conducted barium x-ray of the stomach and duodenum is a little cheaper, causes less discomfort, and is more readily available in some areas. The dyspeptic and his physician should decide what course to take. When the trial of therapy is chosen, both patient and physician should agree to reassess at the end of the trial. Nevertheless, if a patient gets persistent dyspepsia, he may want to know what he is dealing with off the bat.

As discussed previously, there is controversy regarding the importance of gastritis and *Campylobacter pylori* in nonulcer dyspepsia. Many sufferers will have mild gastritis on biopsy. However, as of this writing, the presence or absence of gastritis, or of the organism, has no treatment implications, so a biopsy is not indicated. In the exceptional case, there may be confusion between dyspepsia and other upper gastrointestinal disorders. Patients with pain that might be due to gastroesophageal reflux may need to have an esophageal acid perfusion test (see Chapter 10). If carcinoma of the pancreas is suspected, ultrasonography or CT scan may be done, followed by more sophisticated procedures, such as endoscopic retrograde-cholangiopancreatography (ERCP)—an injection of dye into the pancreatic duct with x-ray. Unless severe episodic pain characteristic of an impacted gallstone occurs, ultrasonography or gallbladder x-ray is not indicated (Chapter 22).

It should be emphasized that a careful history is the most important diagnostic test for dyspepsia and, in the majority of instances, should exclude all but peptic ulcer. The presence or absence of ulcer may only be determined by x-ray, or preferably endoscopy.

TREATMENT

General

It is one of the paradoxes of modern medicine that upon endoscopic discovery of a benign peptic ulcer, the physician and, ultimately, the patient are relieved. Both know or will learn that after 6 weeks of treatment with any of several powerful antiulcer medications, 80 percent of ulcers will be completely healed and symptoms will be gone. The success of the therapy is enhanced if the ulcer patient stops smoking. If the ulcer recurs, no further tests are required, and the treatment is simply repeated. No such easy satisfaction results from failure to find an ulcer in the dyspeptic. There is no drug that is effective here beyond the placebo effect, and symptoms often will not go away. Certainly, much more time is required to search out factors that may be contributing to the discomfort.

Reassurance is the most powerful therapeutic weapon. As in all functional disorders, a person may become worried that serious disease, such as ulcer, gallstone, or even cancer, is present. For many people, the knowledge that this is not the case is all the treatment that is required, and the symptoms either disappear or become less important in their life.

Next, the physician should examine the patient's situation for those contributing factors that can be controlled or stopped, including improper eating habits, smoking, air swallowing, and alcohol consumption. A physician may also help a patient to discover improper coping strategies, or may even detect depression or anxiety of which the patient may be unaware. Some situations cannot be changed easily. Stressful life situations, medications for other diseases, childhood experiences, even an adult's personality are all inevitably part of life; but recognition, nevertheless, is the first step toward adaptation.

Drugs

There is no scientific justification for the use of drugs in the treatment of nonulcer dyspepsia. Normally, there is no excess gastric acid production, break in the upper gut mucosa, or demonstrable motility disorder, so drugs to correct these phenomena make no sense. No agent has consistently been shown to be better than placebo, and most clinical trials are seriously flawed (see

Chapter 21). Yet, in almost all clinical trials of potential dyspepsia drugs, between 25 percent and 60 percent of subjects repond to the placebo. So why not use a drug for its placebo response? Why not indeed—provided it is cheap and perfectly safe? Many people feel better when they take something for their distress.

Am I not spoiling the placebo effect by discussing it? I do not think so. The use of placebo does not imply deception, and it may work even though the taker realizes his drug is a placebo. Experts say a placebo provides an element of control for the individual over his symptoms. What I wish to caution against is the illogical long-term use of costly systemic drugs none of which is perfectly safe, and which may have unpredictable long-term effects. For more discussion of placebos, see Chapter 21.

Because antiulcer and related medications are so frequently prescribed, the reader, at this point, may benefit from a brief review of the drugs that are discussed in Chapter 10. These drugs are valuable in the treatment of peptic ulcer or other organic diseases. But since the pathophysiology of nonulcer dyspepsia is unknown, no rationale for drug therapy exists, and the wide use of these agents without a precise indication is regrettable.

Antacids may constitute the most ideal placebo. Although acid plays no role in the genesis of nonulcer dyspepsia, the side effects of antacids are few and they are safe and readily available. So long as diarrhea does not result, an aluminum magnesium antacid, such as Maalox, may be useful. Unlike antacids, the H_2 blockers, such as cimetidine, ranitidine, and famotidine, are absorbed and do have systemic effects. We have the most information about cimetidine (Tagamet), which has been available since 1977. Although the side effects of this drug are few, it cannot be considered perfectly safe. Further, anticholinergics that tend to delay gastric emptying cannot be expected to improve the dyspectic condition. Even the use of the modern anticholinergic pirenzepine, which primarily reduces acid secretion, makes no sense in nonulcer dyspepsia.

Although sucralfate and the bismuth compounds are not absorbed, they may be safer (but no less costly) than the systemic medications already mentioned. However, since there is no break in the mucosal integrity in nonulcer dyspepsia, mucosa-protecting drugs, such as sucralfate, would provide no benefit despite one marginally successful but flawed trial. As mentioned, bismuth may rid the stomach of *Campylobacter pylori*. One trial has suggested that if bacteria are present, dyspepsia may improve when the patient is treated with a bismuth compound (eg, DeNol, which is available only in the UK; Pepto Bismol). So far, the use of bismuth or antibiotics for this organism does not appear to have a primary role in nonulcer dyspepsia, but they might be tried in difficult cases that also have gastritis. Excessive use may result in bismuth toxicity.

There may be a subset of nonulcer dyspepsia patients who also have delayed gastric emptying. In resistant cases, a short trial of one of the gastrokinetic agents may be reasonable. But here again, the physician should be aware of the possible long-term effects of systemic medication. Metoclopramide (Maxeran), the only gastrokinetic available in the United States, has too many side effects for use in a benign condition. However, domperidone (Motilium), which is available in Canada, seems safe enough.

Simethicone, a surfactant that rids the gut of gas bubbles, is probably of little benefit in getting rid of gas. Nonetheless, it is safe and is not absorbed and might serve as a logical placebo in the person who complains of dyspepsia and flatulence.

SUMMARY

Nonulcer dyspepsia is a common, chronic disorder consisting of epigastric pain or discomfort, that is often meal-related, that may lead the physician to suspect the presence of a peptic ulcer. One-third of patients with such a history will turn out not to have a peptic ulcer, and the distinction may be made only by endoscopy. Because the pathophysiology of this syndrome is not known, there is no rationale for corrective therapy, and drugs have not been proven to be of benefit. Reassurance that no ulcer or other severe disease exists is the cornerstone of management. Sufferers of nonulcer dyspepsia are advised to avoid known contributing factors, such as dietary indiscretions, alcohol, tobacco, and drugs. As with other functional disorders, dyspepsia, or at least the awareness of dyspepsia, may reflect the sufferer's emotional state or adaptation to stress.

CHAPTER TWELVE

"Burbulence"

Symptoms Attributed to Gas

How do I feel today, I feel as unfit as an unfiddle, and it is the result of a certain turbulence in the mind and a certain burbulence in the middle.

Ogden Nash, "New Year's Day 1964"

Although very likely Nash was describing a hangover, it was Sir Avery Jones, the author of a textbook of gastroenterology, who proposed the term *burbulence* to describe the various windy syndromes. Burbulence has a certain cachet that is not conveyed by such terms as gas, burping, belching, bloating, or flatulence. Burbulence nicely describes symptoms arising, or that are thought to arise, from gas in the gut.

EARLY STUDIES OF GASTROINTESTINAL GAS

Air swallowing is called *aerophagy*. The first description for aerophagist was recorded in 1813. He was a conscript, who, perhaps anticipating the battle of Waterloo, practiced the art to avoid service in the French Army. In 1816, Magendie introduced the science of flatology (the study of flatus) by examining gas in the intestines of newly executed criminals. He was able to identify carbon dioxide, nitrogen, and methane. Today, the abolition of capital punishment has necessitated more sophisticated methods of gas specimen collection.

In 1823, Robert Graves, a physician famous for his description of thyroid disease, claimed that the stomach had the power to secrete air as well as acid, and "proved that in dyspepsia this power is morbidly deranged in such a manner as to give rise to a supersecretion of acids and air." Ninety years later, a book appeared with the alarming title of *Flatulence and Shock*. The author, F. G. Cruickshank, reasoned that gastric air secretion, or "pneumatosis," was the only possible explanation for patients (including himself) who suffered spontaneous flatulence and eructation (belching). Although the ability of some patients to generate prodigious amounts of gas continues to amaze, no one now believes in pneumatosis (see Thompson, 1979).

The normal human gut contains 100 to 200 milliliters of gas. J. F. Fries, in 1906, using a rectal tube, recorded that a subject produced 1 liter of gas per day. With more elaborate techniques, other researchers have found that in 24 hours flatus production averages 2 liters. Carbon dioxide, hydrogen, and nitrogen are present in all samples, and oxygen is present in most. Methane and hydrogen sulfide are absent in nearly half of the flatus specimens. It is of passing interest that the normal individual emits 50 to 500 milliliters of gas 13.6 times in 24 hours.

SOURCE OF GAS

The two principal sources of intestinal gas are swallowed air and gases that are produced within the gut (Figure 18). The relative importance of these two sources is variable, but, for practical purposes, gas that is brought up is air, whereas that rumbling in the lower region is usually produced locally. Some gas may diffuse from the blood into the gut lumen.

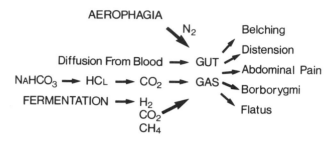

Figure 18.   Sources and symptoms of gas.

Aerophagy

The newborn infant is gasless until its first breath, after which air begins to appear progressively down the gut. At any level, congenital obstruction prevents the distal appearance of air and causes proximal accumulation. Thus, with the infant's first breath is dated not only loss of innocence but also the onset of burbulence. Whether we are aware of it or not, air swallowing and gas in the gut, like sin, are with us unto death. With regular inspiration, the normally negative intraesophageal pressure falls further. Forced inspiration against a closed glottis may suck air into the esophagus. In 1895, this mechanism was described by an Edinburgh physician, J. Wylie, who may have noticed the phenomenon in a bagpipe player. Air that is drawn into the esophagus in this way can be forced up, as intraesophageal pressure is increased with expiration. This art is often mastered by adolescents who delight in demonstrating their burping prowess to peers. Further, individuals who have had their larynx removed because of cancer learn to ingest air in order to generate esophageal speech. The habitual aerophagist may be quite unconscious of the act, and it may not be obvious to the disinterested observer. Nonetheless, what comes up must first have gone down.

Some air may reach the stomach in this manner, and some is swallowed with food. Even without food, 5 milliliters of air accompanied by saliva is ingested with each swallow. A few people gulp air as a nervous tic—a trait often portrayed by cartoonists whose heroes "gulp" when faced with a crisis. Among patients undergoing serial x-ray examinations of the abdomen, those who are nervous are observed to swallow and accumulate more air than those who are not. Occasionally, an individual may swallow air during sleep by inspiring against a closed glottis with a relaxed upper esophageal sphincter.

The composition of stomach gas is similar to that of the atmosphere, and contains 20 percent oxygen. Because the carbon dioxide pressure of blood is higher than that of air, some diffusion into the stomach occurs. Stomach volume increases by 5 percent to 10 percent as swallowed room air is heated to body temperature. Carbonated beverages are an obvious source of gastrointestinal gas, and gusty belching is familiar background music in a barroom. Rapid, gulpy eaters trap air with their food. Gum chewing, thumb sucking, and poorly fitting dentures can also cause excessive production of saliva which must be swallowed. Repeated swallowing also occurs with a postnasal drip or a dry mouth.

Aerophagy is a modest contributor to colon gas as well. Air introduced into the stomach during gastroscopic examination often reappears per rectum within 20 minutes.

Intestinal Gas Production

Gas from Bacterial Action

In addition to nitrogen and a small quantity of oxygen, flatus contains varying amounts of hydrogen and carbon dioxide, along with a number of gases not found in air, such as methane. These latter three gases are produced locally by colon bacteria. There is little gas production in the small intestine because the bacterial concentration is low. Intestinal gases equilibrate between the lumen and the blood and are rapidly cleared in the lungs. Thus analysis of expired air provides an accurate measurement of hydrogen and methane in the gut. This flatulence breathalyser has a number of clinical applications that are discussed below.

Nitrogen

As mentioned, nitrogen (N_2) in the colon largely originates from swallowed air. Diffusion from blood occurs because the intravascular partial pressure of nitrogen is higher than that of the gut lumen (see below). It appears that colon bacteria produce some nitrogen from protein metabolism.

Hydrogen

The hydrogen (H_2) of flatus is exclusively the product of intestinal bacterial metabolism and is dependent upon exogenous, fermentable substrates. Therefore, nonabsorbable sugars, such as lactulose, increase breath hydrogen content, whereas nutrients, such as glucose, ordinarily do not.

Lactose, the milk disaccharide, requires the intestinal mucosal enzyme of lactase for digestion into its constituent monosaccharides of glucose and galactose (Figure 19). In lactase deficiency, the intact disaccharide is not digested or absorbed, and reaches the colon, where bacterial fermentation occurs. Two grams of lactose can release 1,400 milliliters of hydrogen. One lactase-deficient patient, after drinking 2 pints of milk, produced flatus 141 times—a statistic that has been submitted to the *Guinness Book of World Records*. Milk withdrawal effected only a partial cure in this individual, who apparently has a gut flora unusually proficient at generating gas. It has been suggested that such a prolific colon lacks hydrogen-consuming organisms (see below).

Some complex carbohydrates (mainly starch and glycoproteins) are incompletely digested and absorbed in the small intestine, and the residue travels to the colon where it is digested by gut bacteria. The released hydrogen may be excreted in the breath. On the other hand, rice flour is efficiently processed by the small intestine, and no residue reaches the colon.

As early as 1621, it was said that "vegetables engender wind and melancholy." Peas, broccoli, brussels sprouts, and cabbage have a certain gassy notoriety. Contrary to popular belief, onions do not have flatulogenic potential. Spurred by public opinion, the

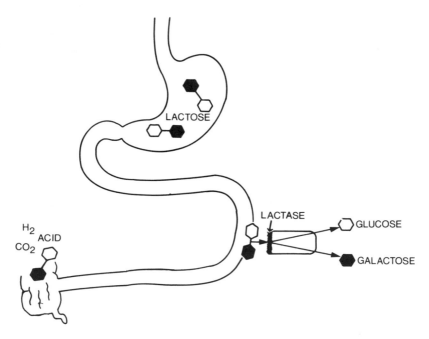

Figure 19.   The digestion and absorption of lactose by the enzyme lactase, which is situated on the luminal surface of small intestinal mucosal cells. Two constituent sugars, glucose and galactose, are released and readily absorbed. If lactase is missing, as in non-Europeans, in certain families, or in a damaged mucosa, the lactose travels to the cecum where it is rapidly destroyed by colon bacteria. The resulting acid stool, small osmotically active molecules, and hydrogen may result in cramps, flatus, and diarrhea. The released hydrogen may be measured in the breath.

bean industry has encouraged research in this area. It was found that beans contain a "flatulence factor" consisting of the complex saccharides stachyose and raffinose. These saccharides cannot be absorbed by the intestine because the enzymes necessary for their digestion do not exist in humans. However, one creature's flatus is another's fulfillment. Certain colon bacteria are capable of metabolizing these substances, thereby releasing hydrogen, methane, and carbon dioxide.

The production of hydrogen by colon bacteria is subject to

many conditions. As we have seen, rice and beans are dietary substrates that provide minimal and maximal fodder for colon bacteria. An individual's gut flora is as unique to him as his fingerprint. Some individuals have bacteria that are particularly efficient at hydrogen production, whereas others have organisms that consume hydrogen. Antibiotics that selectively kill some organisms might have unpredictable results, depending upon whether those organisms are hydrogen producers or hydrogen consumers. In the United States, Indian immigrants have a higher breath hydrogen than native Americans, most likely because their diet is rich in hydrogen substrates.

Normally, 99 percent of intestinal hydrogen is produced in the colon and about 14 percent appears in the breath. Thus, serial breath hydrogen measurements may be useful in a variety of clinical and research situations. For example, lactulose is a disaccharide that survives the small intestine intact, but it is split into its two constituent sugar molecules by the flora in the cecum. With serial measurements after lactulose ingestion, a peak breath hydrogen may be recorded and the interval is the mouth-to-cecum transit time (Chapter 3). In certain diseases of the small bowel or of the pancreas, a standard meal will result in more colon hydrogen production. For example, the inert pentose sugar xylose, which is normally absorbed in the small bowel, travels to the colon in celiac disease with a resulting increase in breath hydrogen. In individuals who cannot digest the disaccharide lactose and are intolerant of milk, a lactose drink will provoke an increase in breath hydrogen (see Chapter 22).

After a carbohydrate meal, there is an early burst of breath hydrogen. This condition may be abolished with mouth wash or tube feedings, suggesting that some hydrogen is released by the action of mouth bacteria on the carbohydrate. Early peaks may also result from bacterial contamination of the normally sterile small bowel, or the meal-stimulated emptying of ileal contents into the cecum.

If a subject is switched from a normal diet to one in which half of the calories are provided by pork and beans, a sixfold increase in flatus hydrogen results—truly an explosive situation! In a study sponsored by the Idaho Bean Commission, it was found that the hydrogen content of expired air rises 5 hours after a bean meal and remains elevated for several hours. After a 24-hour fast, hydrogen disappears from the breath. Thus, science has confirmed what school children have known for generations: "Beans, beans, the musical fruit: the more you eat, the more you toot."

Pneumatosis cystoides intestinalis is a curious condition in which gas-filled cysts are found in the wall of the gut. The cysts contain up to 50 percent hydrogen. Many such sufferers produce unusual amounts of hydrogen in their colons, but one such patient showed resolution after antibiotics.

The unabsorbable carbohydrate of dietary fiber is digested to some extent by colon flora. Indeed, flatus volume has been linked to crude fiber intake, but there is not a breath of information available on burbulence in Africans on a high-fiber diet. Flatulence is a common observation in Westerners who have eaten baked beans or wholemeal bread. It is curious, however, that the situation improves once the subjects are on a high-fiber diet for some weeks. Presumbly, the gut adapts to fiber with improved motility and altered flora. Because a high-fiber diet is now recommended for a number of disorders, we certainly are bound for a generally more flatulent environment. Perhaps the accusatory looks and mumbled apologies that pass between elevator passengers will, in the future, be replaced by a hearty "Your health, sir!"

Carbon Dioxide

Sodium bicarbonate or baking soda reacts with hydrochloric acid in the stomach to produce carbon dioxide (CO_2).

$$HCl + NaHCO_3 \rightarrow NaCl + H_2O + CO_2$$

Hydro-	Sodium	Salt	Water	Carbon
chloric	bicarbonate			dioxide
acid				

One millimole of hydrogen plus 1 millimole of bicarbonate can release 22.4 milliliters of carbon dioxide gas. Therefore, following

cumulated air. The feeling of gastric distension occurs with little or no change in intragastric pressure. The individual's ability to tolerate air in the stomach varies, and some are known to experience discomfort with normal quantities, which suggests an increased sensitivity to normal gas content. Many patients claim that a good belch may temporarily relieve their abdominal distress, and to this end unconsciously swallow air. Those individuals with heartburn and duodenal ulcers swallow more frequently than those without. An urge to burp sometimes accompanies an inferior myocardial infarction (heart attack). But the act of expelling air may be a counterstimulus with no lasting benefit. Once this habit has been established, however, habitual burping may continue long after the original discomfort has faded from memory.

A person's ability to burp is affected by his or her position. While an individual is upright, some swallowed air may not reach the stomach, because food, which is heavier, leaves the air behind. Air that does reach the stomach collects in the cardia above the gastroesophageal junction, from which it cannot escape. The gastric air bubble stays in place as the stomach empties from below (Figure 20). However, the assumption of the supine position seals the cardioesophageal junction by shifting gastric contents over the cardia. This prevents burping and forces the air to empty into the small gut. In bedridden patients with impaired gastric emptying, this position can be a source of discomfort. In the prone position, the gastric bubble overlies the gastroesophageal junction, and belching becomes possible. Sleeping on the right rather than on the left side also favors eructation.

Most patients are relieved to discover the nature of their air swallowing, but many continue to belch especially during emotional stress. Repetitive sallies to the point of exhibitionism are termed *eructeo nervosa*. This may just be an intractable bad habit, or a manifestation of psychiatric illness.

Bloating and Abdominal Pain

The signs of wind . . . are rumbling, swelling, and wandering pain coming suddenly, and suddenly vanishing, a clear tumour that yields

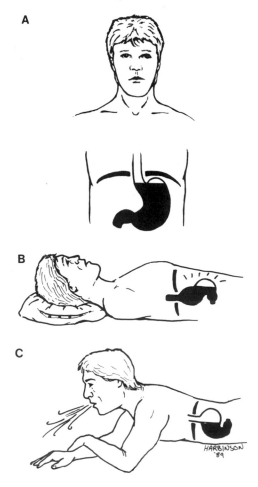

Figure 20.   Effect of position upon the ability to belch. (A) Erect: air that lies in the fundus above the cardioesophageal junction cannot escape. (B) Supine: air collects anteriorly and may not easily be passed distally through the pylorus or retrograde through the esophagus. (C) Prone: air otherwise trapped in the stomach may now escape through the cardioesophageal junction.

to the touch, and that sounds like a drum. Often belching and farting are also signs, and ease after breaking wind usually follows.

J. Feinus (1643)

Many people believe that localized collections of gas cause pain and distension, but this is rarely the case. By infusing the inert gas argon into the gut and measuring its dilution by the intraintestinal gases, it has been demonstrated that patients with burbulence have no more intestinal gas than controls, either when fasting or after meals. The composition and distribution of gas in those suffering from pain are also similar to those of controls. However, those patients with symptoms tend to have longer gas transit time and reflux of duodenal contents into the stomach. This fact suggests that an underlying motility disorder is responsible for the sensation of bloating. The inability to eructate often follows surgical repair of a hiatus hernia. Failure of gastric emptying may result in post-prandial fullness and discomfort, and the sufferer may feel that if only he could belch, all would be well. True distension of the stomach with gas may occur with obstruction of the pylorus by an ulcer, or by conditions that impair gastric contractions, such as the post-operative state, a body cast, or diabetic visceral neuropathy (gastroparesis diabeticorum).

Severe distension of the stomach occurring spontaneously is termed *magenblase* and may be identified by a plain film of the abdomen. This distressful sensation, often accompanied by hiccups, may be misinterpreted as heart or gallbladder pain. Acute gastric distension occurring postoperatively requires decompression with a nasogastric tube.

The *splenic flexure syndrome* is said to result from a collection of gas in the splenic flexure of the colon and is manifest by left lower chest pain. Termed *pseudoangina* by some writers, it does not have the relationship to exercise that one associates with true angina. Such localized trapping of gas, although rarely demonstrated, is sometimes blamed for the *postcholecystectomy syndrome*, but more likely the pain is due to an irritable bowel (see Chapters 13 and 14). Bloating and distension occur in 30 percent of people and are important features of the irritable bowel. Gurglings and rumblings emanate from the abdomen, a phenomenon whimsically termed *borborygmi*. The sounds of insides churning are loudest to the individual himself, and a sensitive person may suffer intolerable embarassment, even when others are unaware of his predicament.

In every human endeavor, it seems there is someone willing to turn another's misfortune into gold. In preparation for the 1976 Olympics, German swimmers had 1.8 liters of air pumped into their colons to improve buoyancy. It apparently helped crawl and backstroke specialists, but a breaststroker complained that the gas-filled gut caused his feet to stick out of the water. Perhaps sports authorities will need to test athletes for flatus, as well as steroids.

Bloating by itself is almost never a symptom of serious disease, but it may accompany other more ominous symptoms. Abdominal discomfort and anxiety, accompanying such gastrointestinal conditions as peptic ulcer, cancer, or gut inflammation, may induce air swallowing and motility changes. Swallowed air is a main source of gas in intestinal obstruction. In celiac disease, chronic pancreatitis, or lactose intolerance, nutrients ordinarily absorbed in the small gut are available for fermentation in the colon. Therefore, a recent onset of burbulence, like any new gastrointestinal symptom, requires vigilance to detect other indicators of serious disease.

Pseudotumor

Distinct from the sensation of bloating is *hysterical nongaseous bloating* described by Walter Alvarez, who worked in the Mayo Clinic in 1930s. Of 150 patients who bloated, he collected 92 whose abdomens became visibly distended in the absence of increased intestinal gas. Described by Robert Bright in 1838, this curious conditon occurs mainly in neurotic female patients, often with such other symptoms as irritable bowel, scanty menstruation, unfulfilled sex, and migraine headaches. An early case may have been Mrs. Weller in Dickens's *The Pickwick Papers* who "always goes and blows up, downstairs for a couple of hours arter tea." Such swelling

has been called *pseudocyesis* (false pregnancy) or *pseudotumor*.
Bright's patient actually underwent surgery for an ovarian cyst,
but none was found. Most patients with this condition assume an
arched position such that, when they are supine, a fist may be
inserted between the spine and the table. Also their diaphragms
are forced downward. The apparent distension may be corrected
by flexing the thighs over the abdomen. On physical or x-ray examination, there is no sign of excess fluid or gas, and the swelling
disappears under general anesthesia without the escape of wind.
The psychodynamics of this curious affliction are difficult to follow,
but horses have been reported to bloat in order to avoid being
saddled!

Farting

> Where're ye be, let ye'r wind gang free.
>
> Robert Burns

Gas that escapes from the nether end of the gastrointestinal
tract has no status in any respectable society. In ancient Rome,
passing gas in a public place was illegal. Those familiar with Chau-
cer will appreciate the fact that making wind has been the subject
of general mirth and private misery at least since the early days of
the English language. In the fifth century BC, one of Aristophanes's
characters complained, "my wind is not frankincense." Thus,
whether gas reenters the world from above or below, it is part of
the human condition. It is indeed fortunate that the upper anal
mucosa has sensors that can distinguish whether rectal distension
is due to gas or feces. Otherwise, farting in a public place would
be more than illegal.

Explosions in the Gut

> Inborn, inbred, engendered in the corrupted humours of the vicious
> body itself, . . . spontaneous combustion, and none other of all the
> deaths that can be died.
>
> Charles Dickens, *Bleak House*

There are several reports of intracolonic explosions resulting from the use of cautery. While electrodesiccating a bleeding point through a sigmoidoscope, an unwary surgeon heard a loud report, and a blue flame shot from the instrument. During subsequent emergency surgery, a rent was discovered near the splenic flexure, necessitating colon resection. In another case, a patient who had been prepared with a 5-liter washout with mannitol suffered a fatal explosion during snare cautery of a polyp. Mannitol may result in bacterial hydrogen production in the colon. The explosive mixture of hydrogen in the air is 5 percent to 75 percent, and that of methane is 5 percent to 14 percent. In 54 patients prepared for colonoscopy by clear fluid diets for 24 hours, castor oil the evening before, and enemas until clear, no explosive mixtures were encountered. Nine hundred individuals prepared for cautery in this manner experienced no mishap. On the other hand, 43 percent of 14 patients with unprepared bowels harbored a colonic bomb. Therefore, it is important that the colon be thoroughly cleansed (not with mannitol) prior to colon electrosurgery. Carbon dioxide must be infused if electrocautery is necessary in the poorly prepared patient.

Those unfortunate persons with gastric fermentation resulting from stasis and low acid content are potential fire hazards as well. One man who had previous gastric surgery happened to belch while lighting a cigarette and suffered burns to his nose and hair. Another person was offered a light by his partner at bridge. Unable to suppress a belch at the crucial moment, he discreetly allowed the gas to escape nasally. Two fan-shaped flames shot through his nose, "just like a dragon, Doctor." Perhaps such individuals should not be firemen or arc welders.

DIAGNOSIS

History

Belching, abdominal distension, borborygmi, and farting may occur alone or along with many of the functional gut syndromes, such as dyspepsia, the spastic colon, or constipation. Although they are not sinister in themselves, the physician should be alert for other historical features that might suggest organic disease, especially weight loss, nutritional deficiencies, or anemia. Scrutiny of the diet may identify culpable substrates, such as beans, brussels sprouts, or lactose. The repetitive burper may be an air swallower and if he can burp on command, the physician may demonstrate to him that he is sucking air into his gullet as a prelude to the belch.

Physical Examination

An abdomen distended with air is tympanitic (a hollow sound when tapped) upon examination. In an emergency situation, it is necessary to distinguish a distended gut from gas in the abdominal space (pneumoperitoneum). This is seldom difficult because the latter occurs in a very ill patient with signs of inflammation (peritonitis). In hysterical, nongaseous bloating, there will be no tympany, and the patient may have an arched back and depressed diaphragm. The distension may be reduced by flexing the thighs over the abdomen. Organic causes of gut distension include obstruction of the bowel or toxic dilatation of the colon that occurs with ulcerative colitis. Accompanying signs in a very ill patient should clearly indicate the root of the trouble. In a supine patient with fluid in the abdominal cavity (ascites) tympany is confined to the umbilical area and should shift as the patient moves onto his side.

In 1905, Walter Cannon felt that the origin of bowel sounds could be determined by their rhythmicity. He identified his own postprandial 3-per-minute gastric contractions. Later investigators have been unable to confirm this finding. Intraluminal air plus fluid are necessary for the gut to produce sound. Most normal bowel sounds, especially those of high frequency, are emitted from the stomach. The colon is responsible for low frequency sounds, and the quietest segment is the small bowel, which contains little air.

A floating stool has long had its buoyancy attributed to increased fat content (steatorrhea), but this is a myth. In malabsorption, unabsorbed substrates allow increased hydrogen and carbon dioxide production, and these gases become trapped in the interstices of the stool. Individuals who are methane producers also report floating stools. Nevertheless, a buoyant stool is a more specific indicator of flatulence than of steatorrhea.

Laboratory

If gastric distension or the rare splenic flexure syndrome is suspected, a plain abdominal x-ray during an attack may confirm the diagnosis. Occasionally, aerophagy may be demonstrated during a barium swallow x-ray.

A lactose absorption test is useful to confirm the suspicion that milk sugar is the cause of gas, especially if the symptoms are reproduced following milk ingestion (see Chapters 16 and 22). However, lactose withdrawal may not completely solve the problem. A stool analysis for fat is sometimes necessary to exclude malabsorption. If a patient is believed to produce excessive flatus, gas collected in a syringe via a rectal tube may be submitted to analysis by gas–liquid chromatography. If the sample is mainly nitrogen, air swallowing is the likely source. On the other hand, detection of large quantities of carbon dioxide, hydrogen, or methane indicates colon fermentation. Due to a shortage of flatologists, such testing is unavailable in most hospitals.

TREATMENT

To discover some Drug wholesome and not disagreeable, to be mixed with our common Food, or Sauces, that shall render the Natural Discharges of Wind from our bodies, not only inoffensive, but agreeable as perfumes.

Benjamin Franklin

As with so many functional complaints, patients may be more worried about the meaning of gas than about the symptom itself.

Therefore, a thorough examination followed by explanation and reassurance is important. Burbulence is part of life, yet there are cultural strictures against its public expression. As mentioned, flatus was a contravention in classic times. Present-day patients should be reassured that a single postprandial belch may be most satisfying and curative. Repeated belching, however, likely indicates aerophagy. Certainly, the passage of flatus must be regarded as physiological, even though there is great individual variation.

The prevention of aerophagy is paramount in the treatment of upper gastrointestinal burbulence. A time-honored remedy for paroxysmal burping is to grip a cork between the teeth. It is impossible to suck air into the esophagus with the teeth parted in this way. Sensitive individuals, however, may find that the cork is as embarrassing as the gas. Biofeedback was used in one group of aerophagists, and each swallow provided auditory feedback through a throat microphone. But the beneficial effect was short-lived.

A postprandial stroll moves the air bubble to the upper stomach in a position to be belched and stimulates gastric emptying. For the nocturnal or bed-ridden imbiber, the prone or left-side-up position facilitates release of air by locating the gastric bubble over the esophagogastric junction (Figure 20). Gum chewers, heavy smokers, and compulsive talkers may notice an improvement when these frailties are forsaken. Loose dentures and postnasal drip in an individual should also receive attention. Finally, small meals eaten with studied slowness can help an individual minimize the gastric trapping of air.

Diet

To eliminate gas, carbonated beverages, soufflés, and whipped desserts should be avoided. Many physicians recommend bicarbonate-containing proprietary preparations to combat gastric acidity and bring up gas, even though their alleged beneficial effect is an unexplained paradox.

To produce gas, intestinal bacteria need a suitable substrate.

If the flatus contains hydrogen, carbon dioxide, or methane, some unabsorbed nutrients must be reaching the colon. The carbohydrates in dietary fiber may be responsible, and, in addition, many people cannot tolerate the high-fiber content of bran, broccoli, or beans. Elimination of fiber from the diet will then starve the gas-producing bacteria. Similarly, in lactose intolerance, withdrawal of milk eliminates a gas substrate.

Another approach to the elimination of gas is to place the patient on an elemental diet that contains predigested carbohydrates, fats, and protein ready for absorption. If gaseousness is decreased, then foods might be added one at a time. A careful record should be kept, indicating which items are responsible for increased symptoms. Of course, the patient could simply starve his flora by fasting, but he might perish first.

Drugs

Antibiotics

Sulfonamides increase hydrogen production following bean ingestion, whereas neomycin has an unpredictable effect. Many sufferers state that their troubles worsen or improve following antibiotics given for various other reasons. The result must depend upon whether gas formers or gas consumers are killed. The results of deliberate tampering with the gut flora by antibiotics are unpredictable, and there may be serious side effects.

Carminatives

Used by Hippocrates, carminatives are among the oldest known medicines. They are extracts of volatile oils that when ingested cause an epigastric warmth followed by a belch that releases gas from the stomach. The best known carminatives are cinnamon, cloves, ginger, and peppermint. The latter commonly flavors antacids and liqueurs, and peppermint candies are often found near the cash register in restaurants. Intragastric intallation of essence of peppermint relaxes the lower esophageal sphincter, and heartburn is sometimes worsened. Most antacid preparations are flavored with peppermint, whose carminative effect may help bring up gas.

Defoaming Agents

Silicone-containing defoaming agents were first employed therapeutically in ruminants suffering from bloat and are sometimes used in human beings. Simethicone is often added to some commercial antacid preparations. Because of its high surface activity, simethicone causes bubbles to coalesce, but whether or not gas is more easily eliminated in big bubbles than little ones is uncertain.

In one experiment, simethicone administered with lactulose in volunteers reduced breath hydrogen when compared to placebo. However, the placebo tablets contained a fermentable filler which itself produced hydrogen. Even if true, the reduction of breath hydrogen by simethicone is unexplained and, as there were no symptoms, the clinical significance is doubtful. In another experiment in 10 healthy subjects, charcoal ingestion reduced the breath hydrogen generated by a plate of beans, but simethicone did not.

In an uncontrolled trial, researchers observed that three quarters of 200 patients with burbulence improved on simethicone taken 4 times a day, but that most subjects redeveloped symptoms when the drug was withdrawn. In patients recovering from surgery, 80-milligram tablets of simethicone administered every 4 hours reduced pain and led to earlier release of gas. In another trial, postoperative distension was also reduced. In spite of these two controlled studies, some researchers remain unconvinced. At least, simethicone's safety seems certain, and it may serve as a harmless placebo. The drug is useful in dispersing froth during endoscopy and barium contrast x-rays.

Antacids

Magnesium and aluminum hydroxide neutralize hydrogen ions in the stomach, rendering them unavailable for reaction with gut bicarbonate. Whether or not this action significantly reduces carbon dioxide release in the duodenum is debatable. Many antacid preparations contain peppermint and simethicone. As in the case of dyspepsia, these drugs may be most useful as placebos.

Absorbents

Kaolin and chalk are said to absorb gases. Patients with flatulence following ileal resection reported improvement while taking the anion-exchange resin cholestyramine (see Chapter 16). This could be due to decreased motility, altered substrate availability, or adsorption of gas by the resin. These substances are all awkward to ingest, messy, and only weakly effective, but they might be worth a try with desperate cases.

Activated charcoal is a fine, black, odorless and tasteless powder. The residue of destructive distillation of organic materials, it is treated by steam at high temperatures to increase its gas adsorptive power. In two studies, capsules of activated charcoal reduced the breath hydrogen rise following the now notorious bean meal. Happily the number of "flatus events" were also reduced. Thus, characoal may be an effective antidote to beans. Alternatively, it may be more simple to burn the beans!

Gastrokinetic Agents

The gastrokinetic agents metoclopramide (Maxeran), domperidone (Motilium) and the investigational drug cisapride stimulate gastric emptying and small gut transit. This result has led to their use in postprandial epigastric fullness, gas and belching, even though no studies address the effect of these drugs on the gas symptoms directly. Metoclopramide has serious side effects and should not be used for such a benign condition (Chapter 11).

Other Drugs

In our drug-oriented, narcissistic culture, the belief is abroad that there is a pharmacologic cure for all the afflictions of human beings. Because the symptoms of burbulence are likely to be prolonged and recurrent, tranquilizers offer little but a dulled mind, and should not be used unless directed against a specific emotional disorder. There is no evidence that fanciful preparations containing pancreatic enzymes (Phazyme) to improve digestive efficiency are of any benefit. Claims for the beneficial gas-clearing effect of compounds containing anticholinergics, tranquilizers, narcotics, and antacids are reminiscent of the eighteenth-century advertisement for Dr. Benjamin Godfrey's "Cordial."

> It is with safety and good success given to the those troubled with burstenness, especially in time of great pain, being very powerful for the expulsion of wind, and that to admiration; it assuages the torment and griping of the stomach and bowels, and drives out the wind both upwards and downwards which is often the cause of griping. (Etherington's *York Chronicle for 1775*, The Castle Museum, York, England)

Dr. Godfrey's concoction contained the narcotic laudanum and was responsible for the deaths of several children. Yet we cannot be smug, because such wanton use of hazardous drugs continues.

BURBULENCE IN THE SPACE AGE

Despite many studies and imaginative remedies, burbulence will be a nuisance for some time to come. However, do not despair, because help is on the way from unexpected sources. Astronauts have been faced with a number of unique medical problems, not the least of which is flatulence (Figure 21). The necessity of prolonged confinement in an unventilated space capsule, which is exposed to varying pressures, has led NASA authorities to study the problem. The bean industry, smarting from generations of innuendo about its product, has been busy as well. Currently, scientists are working on a "clean bean" to thwart the bacterial production of gas.

SUMMARY

Burbulence refers to belching, bloating, gurgling, and farting, all of which are attributed to gastrointestinal gas. Although harm-

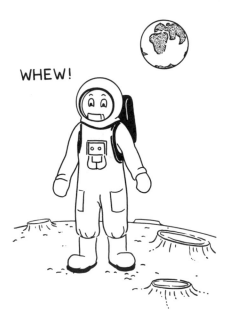

WHEW!

Figure 21.   Burbulence in the space age.

less, these phenomena may lead to social, psychological, and physical discomfort. Burbulence is a fundamental, physiologic, human
problem known since antiquity and has cultural implications in
many societies.

   Air swallowing is responsible for upper gastrointestinal gas.
To some extent, lower intestinal gas may result from air swallowing
or diffusion from blood, in which case the gas is predominantly
nitrogen. More important is the release of hydrogen, carbon dioxide, and methane by the action of bacteria on unabsorbed substrates reaching the colon. Burbulence may occur with or without
increased gas in the gut. Altered gut motility or sensitivity may
explain these sensations. Occasionally, gas symptoms may accompany those of an organic diseae, such as malabsorption or acute
gastroenteritis.

   Prevention of air swallowing may be difficult, but excessive burping or swallowing, carbonated beverages, and poor eating habits should be avoided. Intraintestinal gas production may be prevented in some cases by withdrawing milk, gassy vegetables, or sources of dietary fiber. Simethicone, carminatives, and antacids are useful as placebos. Charcoal, if timed correctly, may reduce breath hydrogen production following a gas-producing meal.

Burbulence is the product of complex interrelationships among ingested air, gut motility, colon flora, unabsorbed substrate, gas-absorption characteristics, and the psyche. We have much to learn before we can bid a final farewell to flatulence.

CHAPTER THIRTEEN

The Irritable Bowel

Our bowels are at their best when they function silently and with only intermittent recognition.

Sherwood Gorbach (1974)

The irritable bowel syndrome (IBS) is an enigmatic and variable constellation of symptoms accounting for 20 to 30 percent of patients referred to a gastroenterologist who devotes much of his time proving that they do not have a more serious disease. Were it not for the IBS, fewer physicians would be required and the diagnosis of organic gut disorders would be much easier. This chapter will emphasize the great prevalence of the IBS, the lack of any reliable pathophysiologic marker or test, the patient's hidden agenda, which may have little to do with physical symptoms, the importance of a positive diagnosis, and Sir William Osler's principle of "do no harm" in investigation and treatment. Because this syndrome is troubling enough, inappropriate tests or treatments can only make matters worse.

DEFINITION

A *functional gastrointestinal disorder* may be defined as a "variable combination of chronic or recurrent gastrointestinal symptoms not explained by structural or biochemical abnormalities. These may include syndromes attributable to the esophagus, stomach, biliary tree, small or large intestines or anus." The *irritable bowel syndrome* is "a functional disorder attributed to the intestines:— abdominal pain;—symptoms of disturbed defecation [urgency, straining, feeling of incomplete evacuation, altered stool form (consistency), and altered stool frequency/timing]; bloatedness (distension)." Although these definitions have been accepted by an international community of gastroenterologists, they are imperfect (Thompson *et al.*, 1989).

The lack of any pathophysiologic marker requires a definition of the IBS according to its symptoms. It is not likely one disease, but many. Even within the IBS definition, some patients will have predominant diarrhea, or pain, or other symptom. Thus the physician must specify symptoms when studying or treating patients.

Perhaps the symptoms or syndromes that we now call *functional* will someday have an organic explanation. For example, before recognition of lactose intolerance, patients with that disorder would have been considered to have IBS. Idiopathic bile salt malabsorption is another organic explanation for symptoms previously thought to be functional. For the present, however, the cause of IBS is unknown.

EPIDEMIOLOGY AND COST

No understanding of the IBS can begin without a knowledge of its astonishing prevalence in the population (Chapter 5). It is well to remember that abdominal pain relieved by defecation and other symptoms characteristic of the IBS occur in 10 to 20 percent of apparently healthy Western adults, most of whom do not consult physicians. Even though the prevalence in both sexes is similar, women are 3 to 5 times more likely to see a doctor than are men. In the Indian subcontinent the opposite is the case.

It is therefore germane to consider why a minority of IBS sufferers seek medical advice, whereas the majority suffer in silence. It is facile to attribute health-seeking behavior to severity of symptoms alone. As we shall see, there are other possible reasons that may be even more important, and their recognition may provide a valuable clue to management.

Psychiatric and personality disorders are more common in IBS patients, yet seem no more prevalent in IBS subjects at large than in normal people. Many subjects date the onset of symptoms, or at least the reporting of them, from a threatening life-event, such as a marriage breakup, a loss of a job, or a death in the family. Heightened awareness of the individual's own mortality may follow the death of a loved one from bowel disease. Thus, bowel disturbance, happily ignored for years, becomes menacingly acute. To make matters worse, relatives and cancer societies urge checkups for any bowel disturbance. Finally, in modern cradle-to-grave welfare systems, there is a growing expectation that no one should suffer, and that there is a pill for every ill. Not only is this expectation an illusion, but its consequences are very expensive.

The IBS is the commonest condition seen by Western gastroenterologists, consuming more of their time than inflammatory bowel disease. The cost of drugs used for this condition is very high despite sparse evidence of their efficacy. There are more sinister costs as well, since IBS patients are liable to undergo unnecessary surgery. The symptoms of IBS are not those of early cancer or inflammatory bowel disease, yet investigations of IBS patients can divert resources from the detection of these more serious diseases. Frustrated with the failure of conventional medicine to abolish their symptoms and perhaps with inadequate attention to psychosocial considerations by their physicians, many unhappy sufferers fall prey to megavitamin protagonists, environmentalists, and other charlatans. If sufferers understand the IBS better, these unnecessary costs can be minimized.

ETIOLOGY AND PATHOGENESIS

The cause and mechanism of the IBS are unknown and, justifiably, the discussion could end here, because the great volume of work described in the following pages only provides glimpses of the truth. Our understanding of functional bowel disease is so rudimentary that future generations will consider our etiologic notions primitive and our therapeutic nostrums naive. Nevertheless, it is important to know the state of the art, for art more than science is the basis of contemporary management. There are hints, too, that the IBS is not just a physical illness. The gut is prone to external influences, as the elegant work of Beaumont, Wolf, and Almy showed long ago (Chapters 2 and 6). Perhaps nowhere in medicine is the interaction of mind and body more aptly demonstrated. If we neglect one in favor of the other, we do the subject a disservice.

This section will deal with the important motility and endocrine observations in IBS patients, and evidence for possible psychological, dietary, and other causes.

Motility

No organ in the body is so misunderstood, so slandered and so maltreated as the colon.

Sir Arthur Hurst (1935)

In the 1960s, several researchers employed intracolonic pressure sensors to demonstrate that resting sigmoid pressure is often decreased in diarrhea and increased in constipation and abdominal pain. It is easy to imagine the sigmoid behaving as a valve or sphincter holding back stool in the constipated (Figure 22). In those patients with diarrhea, a lax sigmoid might allow liquid feces to trickle through the rectum, where it prematurely triggers the defecation reflex. Unfortunately, this neat hypothesis does not stand close observation. For example, recent experiments show more frequent fast contractions in diarrhea-dominant IBS patients than in those patients with constipation. The colon moves in ways too subtle and complicated to be accurately assessed by our primitive methods. The proximal colon and small bowel are even more dif-

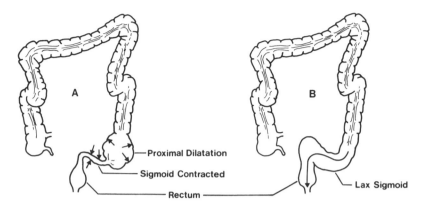

Figure 22.   The sigmoid sphincter. (A) A hyperactive sigmoid holds back stool so that constipation occurs with a few, hard, pelletlike stools in the rectum that are insufficient to trigger defecation. Attempts of the bowel to force feces through causes abdominal pain. (B) A lax sigmoid permits liquid feces to trickle prematurely into the rectum, resulting in urgency and diarrhea. However, this is an oversimplification and clearly, the entire colon and the small bowel are implicated in the IBS. These tendencies are not true in all cases.

ficult to observe yet no doubt play an important role in the genesis of disordered bowel habit and abdominal pain.

By employing breath hydrogen as a measure of mouth-to-cecum time (Chapter 12), some studies have suggested that diarrhea is associated with rapid small-bowel transit, whereas constipation, pain, and distension are associated with slow transit.

Some patients suffer abdominal pain and distension after meals because their eating is accompanied by an exaggerated sigmoid pressure response. This "gastrocolonic response" is mediated by a nerve reflex employing cholinergic neurons and a humoral mechanism (see the section on Fat below). It is suggested that colon contractions cause local obstruction, proximal dilatation, and abdominal pain.

Balloons that are inflated in the rectums of volunteers and of IBS patients produce abdominal pain, urgency, and gaseousness. Although the pain was usually experienced below the umbilicus,

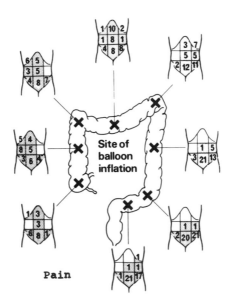

Figure 23.   In 48 IBS patients, balloons inserted by colonoscope were inflated at sites (X) within the colon. In 29 cases, balloon distension of at least one site reproduced the patient's presenting abdominal pain. In many of the remaining cases, the pain was reproduced by balloon distension of the small bowel. The pain was often, but not always, reproduced at an abdominal location adjacent to the inflation site. Reproduced with permission from the *Lancet* (1980;2:443–446).

it could be felt anywhere in the abdomen. Discomfort occurred with less balloon distension in those with the IBS. With the development of flexible colonoscopes, it became possible to inflate balloons at various stations throughout the colon (Figure 23). In 48 patients with the painful type of irritable bowel, the pain could be reproduced in any part of the abdomen, and in 29 of these patients the induced pain was of the same quality and site as the presenting complaint. Many readers will be surprised to learn that distension of the colon can produce pain in the back, shoulders, sacroiliac region, thigh, and perineum. The same research group demonstrated that there are similar trigger points in the small bowel as well. This research reminds us of older work in which distension of the splenic flexure of the colon reproduced chest pain. It is noteworthy that colon distension usually produces pain locally but can do so anywhere in the abdomen and beyond. Although this interesting work confirms the notion that the gut is the seat of the IBS pain, we remain uncertain whether the pain is a normal perception of abnormal motility or an abnormal perception of normal motility. Most likely, both are at work.

Myoelectric Activity

Smooth muscle electrical activity in the rectosigmoid of humans consists of two basic, intermittent slow-wave rhythms: a major one of 6 cycles per minute and a lesser one of 3 cycles per minute. These rhythms appear to originate from the inner or circular smooth muscle layer. Researchers in the United States and in Britain found that the 3-cycle-per-minute activity was greater in their subjects with the IBS than in controls. They later provided evidence that this 3-cycle-per-minute electrical activity was associated with increased 3-cycle-per-minute motor activity, and that this abnormal electrical rhythm persists during asymptomatic intervals.

Contrary evidence appeared when other researchers compared colon contraction and slow-wave frequency in controls, IBS patients with pain, and psychoneurotic patients with no symptoms yet with psychological criteria similar to the IBS group. At one recording site, the number and duration of contractions in IBS patients were greater than in normal subjects, yet by all other motility and electrical criteria, they were alike. The IBS and psychoneurotic groups did not differ significantly from each other by any criterion.

Using a different technology, French investigators recorded electrical activity throughout the colon. They found two types of action potentials: long-spike bursts and short-spike bursts. The former may originate in colon longitudinal muscle, but the latter are action potentials superimposed upon the slow waves originating in circular smooth muscle. In contrast with the slow waves, these spike bursts correlate with mechanical activity in the colon. Short-spike bursts of electrical activity coincided with abdominal pain and were more plentiful in the painful, constipated patient than in controls. In contrast, they were diminished in patients with painless diarrhea.

This area of research will remain confused until the methodology is simplified and standardized. Some studies are done with empty rectums, and others are not. Recording sites and equipment are variable, and diet is not controlled. The exact symptoms of the IBS in most reports are unclear. Patients who enter such studies are highly selected and may not represent the larger number of IBS sufferers who do not consult doctors. Finally, there is no convincing physiological model to explain how the finding of these electrical phenomena can account for the clinical features of the IBS. To date, it must be concluded that the IBS has no physiological marker.

Humoral Factors

Abnormal gut hormone secretion or sensitivity might account for disordered colon activity. Diarrhea occurs in a variety of endocrine disorders, including thyrotoxicosis (overactive thyroid), carcinoid syndrome, islet cell tumors of the pancreas, and medullary carcinoma of the thyroid. Constipation may accompany both hyperparathyroidism (producing high serum calcium) and hypothyroidism (underactive thyroid).

Cholecystokinin (CCK) is a hormone produced in the gut that stimulates the gallbladder to contract. CCK increases colon contractions and reproduces pain when administered to IBS subjects. Although physiologic concentrations of CCK stimulate colon contractions, this hormone does not appear to mediate the gastrocolonic response. Right upper quadrant abdominal pain, which resembles biliary colic in some young women, may be reproduced with CCK injection, even when no gallstones are present. Some researchers propose this procedure as a test for "biliary dyskinesia." However, it is by no means certain that the gallbladder is responsible for the patient's pain. CCK also causes contraction of the common bile duct or intestine.

Motilin is another gut hormone which apparently stimulates myoelectric complexes in the small intestine. Blood levels of motilin increase in IBS patients after stress. Neurotensin stimulates defecation. Adrenal medullary activity (noradrenalin) is increased in "nervous diarrhea." IBS subjects have increased sigmoid sensitivity to parasympathomimetic (cholinergic) drugs, such as bethanechol. One study measured fasting and postmeal concentrations of several gut hormones by radioimmunoassay. All IBS patients had pain, but it was unclear if they had symptoms at time of the study. No differences were detected between patients and controls. As yet, there is no gut hormone profile that will help us identify IBS patients. Any putative role of hormones in the genesis of the IBS is speculative.

The Enteric Nervous System

The enteric nervous system (ENS), or "gut-brain," is the new frontier of gastroenterology. It comprises the myenteric and submucous nerve plexes within the gut wall and their myriad interconnections and ramifications to muscle, submucosa, and mucosa (see Chapter 1). The ENS controls the motor and secretory, perhaps even the immune, activities of the gut. Its associated neurotransmitters, its efferant and afferant nerves, its local reflex arcs, and its connections to the vagus and sympathetic nerves give it a complexity exceeded only by the brain itself. Vagal afferant (to the brain) nerves greatly outnumber efferant (from the brain) nerves, imparting important sensory input to the central nervous system. The vagal and sympathetic connections are the conduit by which activity in the brain can affect the gut and vice versa (see Figure 3).

There are two solitudes in this area of clinical research: on the one hand are the fundamental scientists working with animals who have demonstrated the complexity of the ENS, its neurotransmitters, and its connections to the brain; on the other hand are the clinicians who recognize, categorize, and try to measure gut dysfunction in human beings. Scientific intercourse between these solitudes has been regrettably sparse. Few conferences have attempted to bridge this gap; yet collaboration offers the best chance of understanding the irritable gut.

Possible Causes

As mentioned earlier, a small number of patients with IBS-like symptoms are found to have a physical explanation, such as lactose intolerance. In the following discussion, we will deal with putative factors that may be important in the great majority of IBS sufferers for whom no such explanation is found.

Psychological Factors

It is easy to accept the notion that acute emotion affects gut function. Most people respond to interviews, examinations, or tragedies with a variety of gut symptoms, such as "butterflies," diarrhea, or vomiting. In his classic series of experiments 40 years ago, Thomas Almy demonstrated that acute emotion or stress may alter colon function (see Chapter 7). More recently, British researchers (McRae *et al.*, 1982) used sensors in the small bowel to record the gut's reaction to noxious stimuli. Subjects were required to drive in London traffic or were awakened in the night to demonstrate that stress alters small-bowel motility. It is widely believed that chronic emotion or stress may elicit IBS symptoms in some people. It appears, however, that a given emotion may elicit different responses at different times in different people.

As stated earlier, published work indicates that patients with the IBS are more neurotic, anxious, or depressed than others. Most of these studies suffer from several defects. First, most individuals suffering from IBS complaints do not see a physician. Those who consult a doctor, who are referred to a specialist, and who submit themselves to psychological testing are indeed a small subset of IBS sufferers whose very neurosis may have induced them to consult. We now know that although IBS patients have psychological and personality abnormalities, the majority of sufferers who do not seek medical attention are no different psychologically than normals. Second, few psychological studies attempt to classify the irritable bowel syndrome into subgroups or syndromes that may have different physiologic manifestations. Third, many of the psychological tests used in these studies have not been validated.

During random telephone interviews regarding gut symptoms that were conducted in Cincinnati, subjects were said to have the IBS if they had abdominal pain or gaseous distension and constipation or diarrhea in the previous year without an organic diagnosis (Chapter 5; see also Table 2). Compared with subjects who said they had a peptic ulcer or with the remainder of those who were interviewed, this group had more somatic symptoms, viewed colds and flu more seriously, consulted physicians more often for minor complaints, and were more likely as children to have been pampered by their families when ill. The conclusion appears to be that IBS sufferers are more prone to chronic illness behavior and that this behavior is learned. It may be this behavior that brings many IBS sufferers to the doctor. Such illness behavior may be engendered not only by early life experiences but also by the psychological and personality abnormalities discussed above.

The onset of functional gut symptoms is often preceded by a threatening life-event. Does this indicate that the event triggered the symptoms or that it propelled previously unperceived symptoms to the forefront of the patient's consciousness? The loss of one's parent or sibling because of colon cancer could make an individual suddenly aware of a long-existing cramp. Is the cramp itself a disease? Almy, put the question neatly: Is the irritable bowel syndrome "a qualitative or merely quantitative departure from the psycho-physiologic reactions of normal people?"

Despite the foregoing discussion, we remain uncertain of the extent to which the psychological phenomena observed in IBS patients are cause, effect, or coincidence. Although the importance of attending to the emotional problems of IBS sufferers is unchallenged, it seems that an individual's psychosocial state is not the only factor important in the genesis of the irritable gut.

Dietary Fiber

The stool-bulking effect of bran was demonstrated by several scientific studies performed in the 1930s. However, it was the work of Dennis Burkitt and his colleagues two decades ago that drew attention to the "abnormally" small, slow-moving stools of Westerners compared to those of Africans (Chapter 6). He blamed this on fiber-free, processed foods. The ensuing "fiber hypothesis" attributed many Western diseases to this phenomenon. Constipation and the irritable bowel are said to be rare or nonexistent in Africa. Largely on the assumption that fiber prevents an irritable bowel, bran has become popular as a treatment. Yet bran, which tends to be the chief vehicle of Western fiber, is different chemically from that found in the African diet. Furthermore, from published work, we cannot be sure that the IBS does not exist in Africans.

Despite the beneficial effect of bran on constipation, it seems likely that fiber deficiency is not the sole cause of the IBS, though it may be a contributing factor in many cases. Certainly, a complete and lasting cure cannot be guaranteed solely through fiber replacement. Although fiber increased stool output in a study of healthy volunteers, personality factors were also important determinants (Chapter 3).

Foods and Food Allergy

Occasionally, bran increases IBS symptoms, and the physician rarely encounters a gluten (wheat protein)-sensitive diarrhea that is not due to celiac disease. Because wheat flour is incompletely absorbed in humans, it could account for some symptoms (Chapter 11). Physicians in Cambridge, England searched by means of elimination diets for specific food intolerances. They found that some patients with abdominal pain and diarrhea that were due to the IBS were intolerant to one or more foods, including wheat, dairy products, coffee, tea, and citrus fruits. The authors found no immunologic abnormality to explain these intolerances. The reported diet-testing procedure was lengthy and difficult, and its benefits have not been confirmed by other studies. In most IBS patients, diarrhea is not the predominant feature; therefore, this mechanism might apply only to the diarrhea subgroup of IBS sufferers.

It is a popular misconception that gut symptoms result from "food allergy." "It must be something I ate" says a typical sufferer, and another item is removed from the diet. Some so-called diet specialists or "environmentalists" prey on such beliefs. Although food allergy does exist, it appears to be rare and almost always is accompanied by allergic manifestations elsewhere, such as rhinitis, urticaria, eczema, or asthma. Most IBS sufferers alleged to have a food allergy relapse on a placebo diet. The phenomenon appears to have a psychologic or conditioned rather than an organic origin.

Fat (Gastrocolonic Response)

We need to know more about the effect of food components on the colon. Individuals with abdominal pain after meals may have an exaggerated sigmoid pressure response that corresponds with pain. Myoelectric activity and motility appear to increase concomitantly after meals, and the magnitude of this increase is proportional to the calories in the meal. The postmeal colonic electrical and motor activity is prolonged in the IBS. This response to a meal is due largely to its fat component. An early gastrocolonic response is inhibited by an anticholinergic drug, suggesting that it is mediated by a neural or cholinergic mechanism. Fat also causes a delayed peak of activity that is inhibited by the concomitant administration of protein or amino acids. This late response may be transmitted by a hormone. These observations suggest that an anticholinergic drug, or a low-fat, high-protein diet may benefit IBS patients whose pain predictably follows meals.

Drugs

Drugs are so commonly used in modern life that we cannot ignore their potential to disturb bowel function (see Chapter 20). Antacids, antibiotics, beta blockers, and narcotics may trigger gut symptoms. Many patients use laxatives (see Chapter 19). Anybody suffering with gut symptoms should probably investigate the medicine cabinet.

Dysentery

Some French soldiers who had acquired amoebic dysentery in North Africa in World War I had continuing gut symptoms following their acute illness. In a minority of such cases, an offending parasite persists, but usually stool tests are negative. In their classic study in 1962 of the IBS, Chaudhary and Truelove found that one quarter of patients dated their symptoms from an attack of gastroenteritis. They stated that this subgroup responded favorably to treatment, perhaps because no serious underlying psychologic or physiologic abnormality preexisted. This syndrome is also common in vacationers who acquire traveler's diarrhea from the tropics. In these cases IBS symptoms may continue long after the offending organism has been cleared from the gut.

DIAGNOSIS GUIDELINES

There is a consensus concerning the diagnostic approach to the irritable bowel. The following guidelines are an expanded version of principles that were agreed upon by a 1988 international panel that met in Rome. For reasons that will become apparent, it is important that a positive diagnosis be firmly implanted in the minds of the physician and of the patient on the first clinical visit. The alert physician may make a diagnosis of the irritable bowel by history with a high degree of specificity and sensitivity. But he must establish credibility with the patient through a careful history and physical examination.

History

The panel outlined the following symptom criteria for the IBS:

1. Abdominal pain, relieved with defecation, or associated with changes of frequency or consistency of stool; and/or
2. Disturbed defecation (2 or more of)
   a. altered stool frequency,

Table 13
Symptoms More Likely to Be Found in the Irritable Bowel Syndrome
than in Organic Abdominal Disease

Symptoms	Organic	IBS	Significance[c]
Pain eased after bowel movement[a]	9/30	25/31	$p < .01$
Looser stools at onset of pain	8/30	25/31	$p < .001$
More frequent bowel movements at onset of pain	9/30	23/31	$p < .01$
Abdominal distension	7/33	17/32	$p < .01$
Mucus per rectum	7/33	15/32	NS
Feeling of incomplete rectal emptying	11/33	19/32	NS
	($n = 299$)	($n = 108$)	
A. Abdominal pain[b]	55%	96%	NS
B. Flatulence	50%	85%	NS
C. Irregularity	42%	85%	NS
A + B + C	10%	70%	$p < .0005$
Symptoms more than 2 years	39%	70%	$p < .0005$
Diarrhea and constipation	30%	65%	$p < .0005$
Pellety stools or mucus	38%	76%	$p < .0005$

[a] Adapted from the *British Medical Journal* (1978;2:653–654).
[b] Adapted from *Gastroenterology* (1984;87:1–7).
[c] $p < .0005$, very highly significant; $p < .01$, significant; NS, not statistically significant.

    b. altered stool form (hard or loose/watery),
    c. altered stool passage (straining or urgency, feeling of incomplete evacuation),
    d. passage of mucus;
    usually with
  3. Bloating or a feeling of abdominal distension.

Often there are other upper gastrointestinal, somatic, and psychologic symptoms, at least in those patients seen by the specialist.

Table 13 indicates symptoms that are found to be more common in the IBS than in organic abdominal disease. Also Figure 24 shows how some of this information might be used. Abdominal pain relieved by defecation, abdominal distension, and looser and more frequent stools with pain onset are suggestive individually

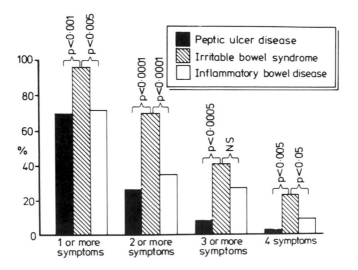

Figure 24. Abdominal pain relieved by defecation, abdominal distension, altered stool frequency, or consistency with pain onset are all individually more likely in the IBS than in organic abdominal disease. The more of these symptoms that are present, the more likely is the subject to have IBS and the less likely to have organic abdominal disease. Reproduced with permission from *Gut* (1984;25:1089–1092).

of IBS rather than peptic ulcer or inflammatory bowel disease. The more such symptoms are present, the more likely is the IBS to be the cause of the patient's complaints. The usefulness of these criteria in positive diagnosis has been confirmed in a Mayo Clinic study.

Of course, IBS symptoms may occur in patients with organic disease. Obviously, such symptoms as weight loss, anemia, blood in the stool, and fever cannot be explained by the IBS and require further inquiry. Bright red blood on the outside of stool may be due to hemorrhoids or a fissure (anal tear). Long-standing symptoms in a well-nourished patient with no family history of gut disease are reassuring. IBS sufferers are no more and no less liable to serious disease than those who do not have the syndrome.

Most IBS sufferers do not present their symptoms to a physician. In Western clinics most patients are women, whereas in the Indian subcontinent the opposite is the case, so psychosocial or cultural factors may influence the decision to consult. Therefore, it is of importance to establish why an individual has chosen this occasion to visit a doctor and what are his or her expectations of the visit. Severity of symptoms are unlikely to be the only reason for consultation. Fear of cancer, recent death in the family from bowel disease, and stress at work or home may point to the single most important service the physician can render to the IBS patient: reassurance.

Any drug might affect the gut. Dietary factors, such as excessive use of coffee, chocolate, or alcohol, should be sought. Diet drinks or chewing gum often contain artificial sweeteners, such as sorbitol or fructose, which are laxative. Lactose intolerance may be encountered in individuals who are not descended from Northern Europeans. Remember, too, an irritable bowel might be triggered by an attack of gastroenteritis.

Chronic, nonbloody diarrhea may be more difficult to confidently blame on the IBS because there are so many other causes (see Chapter 15). Many patients experience diarrhea following cholecystectomy or vagotomy or both. Idiopathic bile salt malabsorption has been described which usually responds well to cholectyramine (Questran). Travelers and campers may become infected with the parasite *Giardia*. Malabsorption states, surreptitious use of laxatives, mucous-secreting tumors of the colon, and endocrine disorders may cause diarrhea. If in doubt, a 3-day stool collection may be helpful (see Chapter 22). The physician may be reassured if the daily stool output is less than 200 grams. More than 500 grams of feces per day or an increased fat content may be indications of an organic cause. In many cases, it is urgency, fecal soiling, or even incontinence, rather than diarrhea, that troubles the person. Some sufferers are reluctant to mention these embarrassing symptoms to a physician.

It is unlikely that the spastic type of irritable bowel with abdominal pain, constipation, hard scybalous stool, and the occasional bout of diarrhea will have the same cause as gas, chronic abdominal pain, constipation, or painless diarrhea (see also Chap-

ters 12, 14, 15, and 16). Each type may require a different therapeutic approach; therefore, the physician should determine which
type of irritable bowel the patient suffers from. These considerations become important should the patient not respond to initial
measures.

It must also be established that the patient has no serious mental disturbance. Those patients who see a physician and are referred to specialists may include individuals with psychoses,
depression, or serious anxieties. Their management will not be
discussed here. However, it is important to stress that most IBS
patients owe at least some of their discomfort to their psychosocial
state. We have seen that a threatening life-event is likely to precede
the IBS patient's visit to a doctor. Indeed, the mind and the gut
share more than nerves and hormones.

Other intestinal symptoms that have been associated with the
IBS include headache, backache, globus, pelvic pain, heartburn,
and esophageal pain. There are two ways in which such associations may be more apparent than real. First, two common conditions, such as IBS and headache, must frequently occur together
by chance. Second, patients may be more likely to report other
symptoms than nonpatients. For example, we found that proctalgia
fugax, heartburn, and globus were equally prevalent in nonpatients with or without the IBS, but they appear to be commoner
in patients. Therefore these associations are of little help in diagnosis.

Physical Examination

Physical examination will help exclude organic disease. Other
than the presence of abdominal scars from negative exploratory
surgery, there are few agreed-upon signs of the irritable bowel.
No doubt, examination has a therapeutic effect in itself.

Sigmoidoscopy not only has an important symbolic benefit
(see Chapter 22), but there are also diagnostic benefits to be sure.
Local diseases, such as colitis, mucus-secreting villous tumors, or
anal fissures, may be found. Some feel that the finding of scybalous

stool, sigmoid spasm, or melanosis coli assists in the diagnosis of functional disease. However, the sigmoidoscopy's most important benefit may be the increased credibility that it imparts to the physician. In patients with noncardiac chest pain, the use of a cardiogram and transaminase measurement reassures the patient, lessens symptoms, and returns him or her to work more quickly. The irritable bowel patient may see the sigmoidoscopy in a similar light. This approach is not mumbo jumbo or witchcraft. Methodical examination and authoritative reassurance are vital components of the art of medicine. Thoughtful medical scientists have recognized this truth for centuries (see Chapter 21).

Investigation

The IBS would present little diagnostic difficulty were it not for the fear that the symptoms might represent organic disease. Of course, the IBS does not provide any assurance against coincident organic disease, so the physician must be wary. In the young North American or European patient, inflammatory bowel disease is the main concern. Careful abdominal examination and sigmoidoscopy should detect most cases. If the hemoglobin, white count, erythrocyte sedimentation rate, and temperature are normal and the symptoms are typical of IBS, no further tests may be needed.

In women, painful intercourse or irregular menses might necessitate a gynecologic examination, although pelvic pain in women frequently is due to the IBS. In patients over 40, the risk of an occult colon cancer is such that most physicians will insist upon an air contrast barium enema or colonoscopy at the initial visit. This procedure should be repeated thereafter only if disease is found, if there is a family history of colon cancer, or if the symptoms change. Among patients referred for barium enema, IBS symptoms were similarly present in normal subjects and those with uncomplicated diverticular disease (see Chapter 18). Individuals with diverticula are usually asymptomatic and when gut symptoms do occur, they may be those of a coexistent irritable bowel.

The physician's decision to do further tests may be influenced

Table 14
Prognosis in the Irritable Bowel Syndrome

Author	Number of patients	Years follow-up	Percentage still symptomatic	Comment
Chaudhary, 1962	126	1–10	63	—
Waller, 1969	50	1	88	—
Holmes, 1982	77	6	57	Diagnosis changed in 4
Svendsen, 1985	112	2	—	Organic disease in 3
Harvey, 1987	97	5–8	74	No change in diagnosis (26% severe; no organic)

by the age of the patient, the nature and duration of the symptoms, the region of practice, and the cost, but common sense must prevail. What is not indicated is a shotgun approach with barium enema, gastrointestinal series, small-bowel enema, cholecystogram, intravenous pyelography, and CT scan on every patient with gut symptoms. Not only is the cost and radiation hazard of this approach substantial, but also the lack of precision reflects uncertainty, thereby undermining the patient's confidence in the diagnosis.

PROGNOSIS

The IBS is a benign condition. The prognosis in terms of life expectancy is excellent, but in terms of continued symptoms, the outlook is not so good. Several studies done in Europe indicate that more than 50 percent of individuals with the IBS suffer their symptoms 1 to 10 years later (Table 14). It would appear that children with recurrent abdominal pain are likely to have the IBS as adults. However, it is reassuring that these follow-up studies also indicate that there is seldom a need to change the original diagnosis. These data suggest that not only is the irritable bowel a chronic, benign condition affecting people over long periods of their lives, but also that it is a stable diagnosis infrequently requiring change or periodic tests.

MANAGEMENT

The management of the irritable bowel requires a high degree of understanding by and between doctor and patient. When a patient has an organic disease, such as peptic ulcer or inflammatory bowel disease, the management plan is usually clear. In contrast, the correct treatment of functional disease is obscure. No recog nizable or verifiable anatomic, physiologic, or biochemical disturbance is present, no pathognomonic feature can be expected to turn up on investigation, and no "cure" is forthcoming. Despite a variety of treatments, the condition tends to persist or recur through a lifetime.

The strategy of management that follows exploits what we know about the IBS to comfort the patient with minimal cost and risk, and will be discussed in 3 stages (Table 15). Stage 1, the *first clinical encounter*, is based upon the establishment of a positive diagnosis, a reassurance that no serious disease exists, an explanation of possible mechanisms of the symptoms, and the establishment of a high-bulk diet. Stage 2 consists of a *follow-up visit* to ensure compliance and comprehension and to detect previously overlooked organic or inorganic factors. Stage 3 concerns the *long-term management* of unsatisfied, intractable, or psychologically handicapped patients.

Stage 1: The First Clinical Encounter

Treatment of the irritable bowel begins with a positive diagnosis based on a history and physical examination. Physicians should be sure to take the patient's symptoms seriously. It is unlikely that any doctor has said "It's all in your head," but some

Table 15
The Irritable Bowel Management Strategy

Stage 1: First clinical encounter
          —A positive diagnosis
          —Establish patient's expectations and reason for consultation
          —Reassurance—absence of cancer, benign prognosis
          —Explanation of how symptoms are generated
          —Initiate bran or other fiber therapy
          —Schedule follow-up visit
Stage 2: Follow-up visit
          —Ensure that patient understands the explanation and is reassured
          —Encourage compliance, ie, proper use of bran
          —Develop new strategy if unimproved
          —Consider alternate diagnoses, but resist unindicated tests
          —Select drugs suitable for certain syndromes
Stage 3: Long-term management of the unsatisfied patient
          —Obtain second opinion of esteemed physician in another center
          —Ensure emotional support and continued access to good health care

patients appear to get that message anyhow. Questions during the interview about diet, stress, emotional state, threatening events, cancer fear, and drugs are relevant and help draw the patient's attention to these factors and prepare him or her for advice to be offered later. A thorough examination and crisp, directed investigation reassure the patient that nothing is overlooked. Even if not mentioned by the patient, anxiety about the meaning of symptoms or fear of serious disease are often part of his or her hidden agenda. The patient must be encouraged to discuss and understand such fears so that they can be set aside as soon as the physician feels sufficiently confident to do so.

An explanation of how the symptoms come about may be especially useful to the sufferer. Often the discomfort and bloating may be confined to the upper abdomen, and the patient needs to know that part of the bowel is there and that it could be the source (Figure 23). Description of the pain that can arise from stretching or from spasm of the gut, or discussion of disordered peristaltic and segmenting movements of the gut that cause altered bowel habits may help the patient understand the complexities of the symptoms. Such supportive psychotherapy has long been believed to be important in the management of many medical disorders, although this notion is difficult to prove in such a fluctuating, subjective syndrome as the irritable bowel.

Nevertheless, Swedish physicians have demonstrated that IBS patients treated with 8 sessions of "supportive psychotherapy which could be performed in any physician's office" had less abdominal pain and psychological disability at 3 months (Svedlund et al., 1983). Most importantly, this improvement over the group that did not receive psychotherapy was even more marked a year later. The essential components of supportive psychotherapy are explanation and reassurance based on a positive diagnosis and discussion of the patient's psychological and social situation (see also Chapter 21).

In the United States, Canada, and Britain, most physicians employ bran or other commercial bulking agents as a method of increasing dietary fiber. Although the several controlled trials available do not strongly support the use of bran, they do show that its use does provide some improvement in constipation and, perhaps, relief of abdominal pain (Table 16). All these trials are flawed, because the numbers of subjects studied are small, the dose of bran is frequently inadequate or the duration of treatment is short (see Chapter 21). However, bran seems effective in relieving the recurrent abdominal pain of childhood, and the widespread use of this harmless substance reflects most physicians' belief in its usefulness. Unlike pharmacotherapeutic agents, bran has a plausible thesis behind its use based on the epidemiologic studies of Burkitt (see Chapter 6). Bran is cheap and unlikely to do harm, although some users experience increased bloating or diarrhea. Because IBS symptoms often accompany uncomplicated diverticular disease, bran is useful in these patients as well.

Thus, among the many methods of increasing bulk in the diet, bran appears to be safe and effective. It is also simple for the physician to assess compliance if the patient starts with 1 tablespoonful of bran 3 times a day with meals and subsequently adjusts the dose as necessary. The use of fiber should be a long-term commitment, and the patient should judge its benefit on the basis of changes in

Table 16

Placebo-Controlled Bran Trials in the Irritable Bowel Syndrome and Uncomplicated Diverticular Disease

Author	Number of patients	Fiber (grams/day)	Duration (weeks)	Placebo response (percentage)	Result
Soltoft, 1976[a]	29	14.4	6	69	Nil
Manning, 1977	13	7	6	38	Pain, bowel habit, mucus improved
Brogribb, 1977[a]	9	6.7	12	NA	Improved, especially pain
Ornstein, 1981[a]	58	7	16	NA	Improved constipation; stool weight unchanged
Weinreich, 1982[a]	39	5	52	56	Improved
Cann, 1984	38	9.6	4	NA	Constipation improved
Lucey, 1987	28	12.8	12	71	Nil, stool weight unchanged

[a] Included patients with uncomplicated diverticular disease.

stool consistency and frequency. Those individuals who tend to pass hard stools with much straining may benefit from the softer, bulkier, and more easily passed stools induced by bran (Chapter 6). Once the benefits have been demonstrated, bran and other fiber-containing foods may be integrated into the diet (see Table 7 and 17). Fiber substitutes, such as bran cookies or psyllium (isbaghula in Britain), may be useful in those individuals who are unwilling or unable to take bran.

It is important that the physician arrange a follow-up visit 6 or 8 weeks after the initial one. In spite of his or her best efforts, many patients do not understand what they have been told, or may not fully comply with therapy. In the patient who has not improved, new approaches should be discussed.

Stage 2: The Follow-up Visit

If the patient is improved at the follow-up visit, no further treatment is required; however, he or she should have access to a doctor should the symptoms return or alter. The unimproved patient, on the other hand, may force consideration of diagnostic alternatives. An open mind in the physician is imperative because the IBS sufferer is not immune to organic disease, even though a positive diagnosis may be made with confidence and very infrequently needs alteration. A review of the essential features of the history should be sufficient. Provided that no new information surfaces, the physician and patient should resist the temptation to undertake further investigative procedures, particularly those that extend beyond the lower gastrointestinal tract.

Physician and patient must be satisfied that the bran is being correctly taken, and often more, or more consistent use, of the bran is beneficial. In such instances, the use of raw bran is preferred since compliance can be accurately reported to the doctor. With improved bowel habit, the patient may work fiber into the diet, taking care that the beneficial effect is maintained (Table 17).

An examination of the data presented in Chapter 21 (Table 31) reveals that one third to one half of individuals with functional

Table 17
Some Sources of Dietary Fiber[a]

	Total dietary fiber[b] (g/100 g)
Bread	
White	2.72
Brown	5.11
Wholemeal	8.50
Cereals	
Bran	44.0
All-Bran	26.7
Puffed Wheat	15.24
Wheatabix	12.2
Shredded Wheat	12.26
Cornflakes	11.0
Special K	5.45
Rice Krispies	4.47
Nuts	
Peanuts	9.30
Brazil	7.73
Vegetables	
Peas	7.77
Baked beans	7.27
Broccoli	4.10
Carrots	3.70
Potatoes	3.20
Onions	2.10
Tomatoes	1.40
Fruit	
Pears (fresh only)	2.44
Peaches	2.28
Strawberries	2.12
Bananas	1.75
Apple (without peel)	1.42
Cherries	1.24

[a] Adapted from the *Journal of Human Nutrition* (1976;30:303–313).
[b] Total dietary fiber of selected cereals, vegetables, and fruits. The composition of this dietary fiber, and therefore its effect on colon function, may vary from item to item.

complaints improve on inert medication. An understanding of this placebo response is very important. Whether it represents the natural history of the disease, or reassurance, or some psychologically mediated benefit, there are nevertheless several implications. First, no drug can be deemed useful in a functional disorder without vigorous testing in controlled clinical trials. Such trials and their pitfalls are discussed in Chapter 21. Second, placebos, if harmless, may be useful, and bran may thus qualify. Third, the response to inert substances reminds us of the art of medicine; the therapeutic effect of a successful patient–physician encounter. To date, despite dozens of clinical trials, very few of which are scientifically sound, no drug has proven to be generally effective in the IBS.

Drugs for Certain Indications

There are occasions when the physician might consider the use of drugs for certain specific indications within the IBS (Table 18). For example, in those patients with the diarrhea-dominant IBS, featured by loose, frequent stools and urgency, loperamide (Imodium) may be effective. Often patients with diarrhea suffer incontinence, and the resulting embarrassment may be the most significant disability. Loperamide appears to increase anal sphincter tone, to reduce colon myoelectric activity, and to slow small-bowel transit. Because it does not pass the blood–brain barrier, it is the safest of the opioid (codeinelike) antidiarrheal drugs. Loperamide might also be used if the patient anticipates a diarrheal attack at the time of an important engagement. Further, in diarrhea-dominant IBS, cholestyramine (Questran) might rarely be of help, because it appears, in this case, that the ileum fails to reabsorb endogenous bile salts (Chapter 16).

For over 35 years, anticholinergics have been the most extensively studied class of drugs in the treatment of the irritable bowel. Reviews of the studies in 1972, 1975, and 1988 concluded that benefit was unproven. Newer anticholinergics are available, but it is unlikely that they offer any therapeutic advance. Certainly, claims that profinium or dicyclomine are more specific for the gut with less anticholinergic side effects elsewhere are unsubstantiated.

Table 18
Drugs Useful for Certain Difficult Irritable Bowel Symptoms

Indications	Dose
Diarrhea-dominant IBS	
Loperamide (Imodium)	1 to 2 tablets tid[a] maximum
Cholestyramine (Questran)	1 tsp (4g) tid maximum
Pain-dominant IBS	
Postmeal abdominal pain	
Dicyclomine (Bentylol)	10 to 20 mgm ac
Chronic pain syndrome	
Amitryptaline (Elavil)	Individualize
Peppermint oil	Placebo
Constipation	
Bran	1 tbsp tid + adjust
Psyllium (Metamucil)	1 tbsp tid + adjust
Gas	
Simethicone	1 to 2 tablets tid

[a] tid = three times per day.

Since the pathophysiology of the IBS is not established, it is difficult to interpret studies showing that anticholinergics suppress colon contractions. Nevertheless, the patient who has predictable abdominal pain after meals may benefit from an anticholinergic administered before meals (see the section above on Motility). The object would be to ensure maximum anticholinergic blockade at the time symptoms are expected and minimum exposure to side effects. As mentioned earlier, a high-protein, low-fat diet might be just as effective (see Chapters 20 and 21).

A few patients appear to be obsessed with abdominal pain or other severe symptoms. Relatively small doses of tricyclic antidepressants seem to be effective treatment for some. Antidepressants may provide a remission even though the physician cannot with certitude determine if depression is present. The benefit of these drugs may be due to their antidepressant, pain-killing, or anticholinergic properties.

Calcium channel blockers reduce colonic motility and myo-electric spike potentials following meals (see Chapter 20). If one believes that this activity is important in the genesis of IBS symptoms, then the physician might rationally test their benefit. Two small clinical trials of these drugs were not encouraging, and they suffered many design faults.

There has also been some initial excitment about the smooth muscle relaxing effect of peppermint oil in the treatment of the IBS. However, controlled studies are small and show conflicting results. Peppermint oil does appear to be harmless enough, although the physician should recall that it relaxes the lower esophageal sphincter and may precipitate heartburn (Chapter 10).

Such tranquilizing drugs as the benzodiazepines (eg, Valium) ought to be reserved for anxiety, because there is no evidence to support them as a primary treatment of the IBS. It is worth emphasizing that the IBS affects a patient for long periods, and no drug, especially a tranquilizer, should be considered a long-term solution.

Of those patients who are unimproved on the follow-up visit, some will not achieve satisfaction. Much patience is required of patient and doctor. Time is necessary for encouragement, discussion, and reassurance since the need for these is great. Certainly, access to continuing medical care is important, and the patient should resist the temptation to doctor shop, or seek the care of unconventional practitioners.

Stage 3: Long-Term Management of the Unsatisfied Patient

Despite much treatment effort, the IBS patient may remain unsatisfied, and this situation can challenge both the sufferer's patience and the physician's skill in dealing with anxiety, depression, and often hostility. Here, more than in many situations, a good physician–patient relationship, especially of trust, is necessary to provide the support that such a patient needs.

In the event that the physician–patient relationship deteriorates, the physician may wish to consider certain referral options. If the patient is emotionally ill, psychiatric consultation may be useful and should be willingly agreed to. However, most IBS patients neither need or profit from such referral. Although biofeedback is effective in some patients with fecal incontinence, its benefit to the other, more prominent features of the IBS has not been demonstrated under controlled conditions. An elimination diet might be tried, especially in patients with diarrhea. However, other than in the experiment that was done in Cambridge, England, the results do not seem to justify the effort. One group of investigators demonstrated the superiority of hypnosis over placebo in resistant cases. However, this study was not blinded and needs confirmation.

If the patient begins to lose confidence in the physician, he or she may find it useful to obtain a second opinion. The consultant, ideally in another medical center, will usually reinforce the diagnosis and endorse the plan of management. This may make the patient's relationship to the primary physician and subsequent care easier. Beyond this, doctor shopping for a "quick fix" is costly, harmful, and futile.

SUMMARY AND CONCLUSION

The IBS is a chronic, relapsing functional disorder attributed to the small and large intestine. The symptom complex includes abdominal pain, altered bowel habit, and abdominal distension along with several associated symptoms. The cause and mechanisms are unknown. Although some abnormalities of small and large gut motility and electrical activity have been described, none is sufficiently specific or sensitive to serve as a diagnostic test. Psychologic factors are common in that minority of sufferers who see doctors, but not in those who do not. It seems likely that the syndrome is a result of many factors. The variable but dramatic effects of acute mental and physicial stress on the gut have been documented. Lack of dietary fiber is important. Gastroenteritis, drugs, stressful life-events, or other environmental situations seem to be triggering factors. Since there are no acknowledged signs or tests for the syndrome, it must be diagnosed by symptoms. Usually, a positive diagnosis may be made with confidence on the first clinical encounter.

Since this is a chronic, benign disorder with no important sequelae, and since no agent is proven effective, management strategy should be based on the available data and common sense. An early, confident, and positive diagnosis and recognition of the psychosocial or worry factors that may underlie the patient's visit can serve as a platform for reassurance, and can be the doctor's most important therapeutic weapon. This strategy may be supported by a sympathetic hearing of the complaints and an explanation of where and how the symptoms arise.

Bran or other bulking agents are often prescribed by most physicians. Bran is effective for constipation and may at least achieve a placebo response without harm or cost. There are many arguments against the use of drugs in the irritable bowel. Specific drugs might be recommended for diarrhea, constipation, gas, or pain in certain circumstances, but they are no substitute for the steps outlined in this chapter, and the provision of reassuring continuing care as necessary.

In a benign condition that affects 10 to 20 percent of people, physicians cannot apply the usual patient care paradigm. Economical, safe, circumscribed investigation and attention to psychosocial or life-style factors must take the place of a pharmaceutical quick fix. We do not yet know whether the IBS is a disorder or a series of disorders of physiology that are liable to correction, or whether, like tears, IBS symptoms are simply a means by which our bodies respond to our environment. For the present, we should heed the advice of those great twentieth-century physicians—Osler, Hurst, and Almy—and see that we do no harm.

CHAPTER FOURTEEN

The Chronic Abdomen

Chronic, undiagnosed abdominal pain may pose difficult and frustrating problems in diagnosis and management. Imprecise diagnosis is disappointing to both patient and physician. Terms like "abdominal pain not yet diagnosed," "functional," or "psychogenic abdominal pain" may sustain the physician's mystique but may do little to clarify the cause or indicate useful treatment. Patients seeking help for chronic pain risk two harmful extremes of management. In one extreme, the physician, unable to understand the nature of the complaint, may minimize its importance and force the patient to seek advice elsewhere. Regrettably, there are charlatans who prey on such patients. At the other extreme, repeated complaints of abdominal pain may generate costly consultations, hazardous investigations, and futile treatments (even surgery), which serve only to exaggerate the importance of the pain and the patient's concern. The chronic abdomen is the most difficult gut reaction to understand or treat.

In many or most cases, the gut is the suspected site of the pain, and some evidence of gut dysfunction may be detected. Thus, the chronic abdomen is a syndrome of the irritable gut. It should be remembered that there are other abdominal organs that could be a source of pain, and there are some instances in which the pain appears to be a manifestation of mental illness. Further, this chapter is not a discussion of the acute abdomen, which is usually handled by the surgeon. Nor will I discuss in any detail chronic recurrent abdominal conditions, such as peptic ulcer or biliary colic, except to differentiate them from the chronic abdomen.

PREVALENCE

The chronic abdomen might be defined as a functional disorder consisting mainly of abdominal pain of more than 6 months' duration that is usually attributed to the gut. We have seen that chronic or recurrent abdominal pain occurs in 10 percent of school children and about 20 percent of adults (Chapter 5). Some of these pains may be due to organic causes, but the majority occur in the absence of any demonstrable pathology. Studies of patients with abdominal pain who were seen in hospital or clinic indicate that 85 percent have no organic cause for their pain. Even 41 percent of patients attending an emergency room were found to have no organic cause (Table 19).

We should be reminded that although many individuals suffer from abdominal pain, most of them do not report it to a doctor. Therefore, the reason that a patient has sought medical advice is important. Often it is not the severity of the pain that troubles the patient but rather fear, depression, or guilt, and these may be important clues to management.

CHRONIC PAIN SYNDROMES AND PSEUDOSYNDROMES

Syndromes

The chronic abdomen is one of the syndromes of the irritable gut, and chronic abdominal pain is the dominant feature. However, there are a number of recognizable syndromes and pseudosyndromes within the chronic abdomen that may have different causes and treatments (Table 20).

Table 19
Functional Abdominal Pain[a]

	Author	n	Pain (percentage)	Functional (percentage)
Nonpatient groups				
In the population	Thompson (UK), 1980	301	21	Most or all
	Drossman (US), 1982	789	24	Most or all
	Bommelaer (France), 1986	1,200	14	Most or all
Patient groups				
In the clinic	Gomez, 1977	96	All	84
	Woodhouse, 1977	20	All	85
In the hospital	Sarfeh, 1976	64	All	85
In emergency room	Brewer, 1976	1,000	All	41

[a] Adapted from Barkin V, Rogers A (eds): *Difficult Decisions in Digestion*. New York, Yearbook, 1988.

Table 20
Chronic Functional Abdominal Pain Syndromes

Syndromes	Pseudosyndromes
The irritable bowel	Splenic flexure
Gas	Celiac artery
Nonulcer dyspepsia	Adhesions
	Biliary dyskinesia
Pelvic pain	Postcholecystectomy
Abdominal woman/man (pain-prone)	Chronic appendicitis
Münchhausen's	Diverticular pain

The Irritable Bowel Syndrome (IBS)

From the irritable bowel discussion in Chapter 13, we have seen that, in most patients, alterations in bowel habit are prominent, and the diagnosis presents no problem. When the abdominal pain is the main complaint, the other features may not be obvious. Careful attention to historical details that connect the pain with bowel function, such as "defecation-related pain," should permit a diagnosis of the IBS.

Gas (Burbulence)

Sufferers of gas seldom call their discomfort a pain (Chapter 12). Bloating, fullness, postprandial abdominal discomfort, usually accompanied by belching, borborygmi, or gas per rectum, lead the sufferer to feel he is full of gas. As we have seen in Chapter 12, intestinal gas is not increased in such situations. By itself, burbulence seldom indicates a serious organic disease.

Nonulcer Dyspepsia (NUD)

For the purpose of this discussion, dyspepsia will be defined simply as chronic, recurrent epigastric pain. Its features, which include a relationship to meals, the relief of the pain with food or antacids, its nocturnal occurrence, its burning quality, or its spring and fall periodicity, may lead the physician to suspect a peptic ulcer. When no ulcer is found, the patient is said to have NUD (see Chapter 11).

Pelvic Pain

Chronic pelvic pain in women without evidence of organic disease is frequently encountered by the gynecologist and is the most common indication for laparoscopy (examination of the abdominal cavity with a viewing instrument inserted through the abdominal wall). In some cases, the pain is associated with menstruation, ovulation, or intercourse, and the phenomenon has been linked, without controlled study, to congested blood vessels in the pelvic organs or pelvic varicose veins. Many such patients are suffering from the IBS and have historical features that link the pain to bowel dysfunction. Pelvic pain is often attributed to anxiety and depression, but the matter has not been studied in any systematic, controlled manner.

The Abdominal Woman (or Man)

A small number of patients have chronic abdominal pain that is unassociated with any bodily function. The pain, which is often described in colorful phrases, is alleviated by nothing and clearly dominates the patient's life. Sixty years ago, Hutcheson described the doctor's dilemma with such a patient, whom he called *the abdominal woman:*

> Incessant demand for sympathy and understanding makes the abdominal woman a veritable vampire, sucking the vitality out of all who come near her. Half an hour with her reduces her doctor to the consistency of chewed string and is more exhausting to him than all the rest of his daily visits put together, for she is always discovering fresh symptoms, will not admit to any improvement in her condition, and has an objection to everything that is proposed.

Such chauvinism is inappropriate because there are also "abdominal men." Male or female, such pain-prone patients challenge the physician–patient relationship and test the physician's resolve to avoid further tests, drugs, or even surgery (Chapter 7).

Münchhausen's Syndrome

This eponym is derived from the legendary eighteenth-century German army officer, Karl Friedrich Baron von Münchhausen, who was noted for his tall tales of the Russian campaign. Typically, patients with this syndrome have bizarre medical and personal histories. The Münchhausen patients' fantastic histories often center on abdominal pain that may lead to costly and hazardous investigations and fruitless surgery.

Pseudosyndromes

A number of chronic pain syndromes can be described that seem to infer causation. Since they mislead or encourage inappropriate management, their unsubstantiated etiology should be stressed.

Splenic Flexure Syndrome

Gas trapped in the splenic flexure is said to generate pain in the left upper abdomen or even in the chest. Frequently, such a mechanism is proposed for anginalike chest pain or postcholecystectomy pain. This phenomenon occurs rarely, if at all. It should be possible to demonstrate a dilated splenic flexure during the pain but seldom is this the case. Although distension of the splenic flexure may reproduce the pain, this is a manifestation, perhaps, of a hypersensitive gut, and is best regarded as a variant of the IBS.

Celiac Artery Syndrome

Intermittent epigastric pain has been attributed to compression of the celiac artery by the ligaments of the diaphragm and is treated by cutting the ligaments. However, the follow-up is short-term, and no physiologic abnormality has been demonstrated which is corrected by surgery. We cannot be certain that compression does not occur in asymptomatic individuals. Thus, a sham operation might be as effective as the division of the ligament. This proposed syndrome should be distinguished from the apparent duodenal obstruction by the superior mesenteric artery. The latter phenomenon is uncommon and likely to be due to chronic intestinal pseudo-obstruction. It will not be discussed further.

Adhesions

"Adhesions," the exhausted cry of the diagnostically destitute, are often blamed for the chronic abdomen. No doubt adhesions are a cause of acute bowel strangulation, which is a surgical emergency, but their importance in chronic recurrent abdominal pain is doubtful. It is well known that patients with the IBS are prone to surgery in which no pathology is found. Symptoms following such surgery may continue to be those of the IBS. Women with chronic pelvic pain are no more likely than other women with infertility to have adhesions discovered when their abdomens are examined through a laparoscope. The distinguished British surgeon, Alexander Williams, has stated that he believes "it to be a poorly substantiated myth that adhesions can cause abdominal or pelvic pain." Anybody who claims miraculous cures after lysis of adhesions "should be aware of the powerful placebo effect of the procedure."

Biliary Dyskinesia

Some patients with a normal gallbladder and bile ducts and no stones have recurrent attacks of upper abdominal pain resembling biliary colic (gallbladder attack). As in the gut itself, balloon distension of the common bile duct produces pain in the epigastrium, the right hypochondrium, and sometimes the back—a distribution similar to that of biliary colic. The characteristic abnormalities of biliary dyskinesia are said to include an elevated *sphincter of Oddi* (SO) pressure and even retrograde peristalsis. Although this seems to be an entity, great caution is needed in interpretation of the pain or the SO pressure recordings. Most patients with such pain do not have SO abnormalities. Indeed, 21 of 22 patients with stoneless or removed gallbladders and extensively investigated recurrent upper abdominal pain had the symptom reproduced exactly by small-bowel balloon distension. In such cases, focus on the biliary tree is misplaced.

Postcholecystectomy Syndrome

Distinct from the biliary colic/dyskinesia syndrome is dyspepsia associated with gallstones. This epigastric distress is more or less constantly present, whereas biliary colic occurs in discrete attacks. It is often described as bloating, burning, or indigestion. However, fatty food intolerance and dyspeptic symptoms are no commoner in those individuals with or without gallstones (Chapter 11). Among patients referred for cholecystogram (gallbladder x-ray), dyspepsia was equally prevalent whether stones were present or not. Therefore, a patient with such symptoms can expect no relief with cholecystectomy (removal of the gall bladder). Thus, the postcholecystectomy syndrome implies that the operation was done for incorrect reasons in the first place.

Chronic Appendicitis

Continuous or recurrent right lower abdominal pain may convince a sufferer that he or she has chronic appendicitis. However, appendices removed for this diagnosis are as likely to be normal as those removed incidentally at hysterectomy. Sixty to 90 percent of appendices removed from young women with right lower abdominal pain are normal when examined by the pathologist. In 1940, Walter Alvarez stated that of 255 patients who had previously undergone appendectomy *without* an attack of acute appendicitis, only 2 were cured of their chronic abdominal pain. Sixty-seven percent of 130 who had true acute appendicitis were cured. Thus the chronic appendix is indeed a pseudosyndrome.

Painful Diverticulosis (Diverticular Pain)

A perforated diverticulum leads to painful complications. However, most of that 50 percent of the older population who have diverticula have no complications (see Chapter 18). Abdominal pain occurs in some but not all people with uncomplicated diverticula. Two studies of patients undergoing barium enema demonstrated no difference in the prevalence of abdominal pain between those with normal x-rays and those with uncomplicated diverticula in the colon. Other IBS symptoms were equally present in the two groups. Thus, when pain occurs in uncomplicated diverticular disease, it is likely to be due to a coexistent IBS. Such a coincidence should not be surprising. Abdominal pain occurs in

14 percent to 24 percent of adults and colonic diverticula in one half of the elderly (see Figure 27). At any rate, it is difficult to imagine how the simple existence of colonic diverticula could cause pain.

CAUSE OF THE CHRONIC ABDOMEN

The cause of the chronic abdomen is unknown. Some researchers claim to understand the mechanism of some of the syndromes, but no view has achieved any substantial support. Putative physiologic or psychologic markers have not been validated. In the following discussion, we will deal with these theories and markers under physiology and psychology, and under factitious pain. Because more research has centered around the IBS, and this is likely the commonest type of chronic abdomen, it will receive special emphasis.

Physiologic Factors

The study of gut motility has many hazards. Although it is now possible to access most of the gut, the technology employed to measure gastrointestinal movements is not standardized. Some studies are done with empty intestines, others are not. Diet and other environmental conditions are not controlled. The exact symptomatology of the patients studied is unclear. Finally, abdominal pain, the IBS, dyspepsia, and, indeed, any of the functional syndromes do not seem likely to have a single mechanism.

The three previous chapters have discussed possible motility disorders underlying dyspepsia, burbulence, and the irritable bowel. Nonulcer dyspepsia has been attributed to a disorder of gastric emptying, yet, in most sufferers, this has not been demonstrated. Discomfort that is due to gas occurs with no increase in gas in the gut lumen. The IBS has been associated with a variety of motor or electrical phenomena in the large and small gut, but none of them explain the symptoms or are sufficiently specific to act as diagnostic markers. We have seen that the abdominal pain of the irritable bowel may be reproduced in most sufferers by the inflation of a balloon at specific sites or trigger points within the large or small bowel. This observation reinforces the notion that the gut is often the site of chronic abdominal pain, but does not settle the afferent or efferent issue. Is chronic abdominal pain a normal perception of abnormal gut physiology or an abnormal perception of normal gut physiology?

Psychological Factors

Abdominal pain does not necessarily infer the presence of structural disease. Therefore, some observers are convinced that it may occur as a result of psychological trauma that may be entirely mental or that might act via the enteric nervous system to alter gut physiology or the individual's perception of physiology.

It is a common experience that acute emotion alters gut function (Chapter 7). Examinations, interviews, or tragedies may be accompanied by a variety of gut reactions, ranging from butterflies in the stomach to abdominal pain. Forty years ago, Thomas Almy demonstrated that emotional or physical distress produces spasm, engorgement, and excessive mucus secretion in the sigmoid colon. Other researchers have confirmed the fact that psychological stress can be accompanied by disturbed large and small intestinal motility or myoelectric activity and that such disturbance may be more pronounced in patients with an irritable bowel. It is not known, however, whether motility changes are mechanisms of pain or epiphenomena.

Although IBS patients have more depression, anxiety, or neuroticism than controls or patients with organic gut disease, most IBS sufferers do not see a doctor for their symptoms. These non-complainers, unlike IBS patients, have a psychological makeup that is similar to asymptomatic people. It may be that the sufferer of abdominal pain is motivated to see his physician by psychological or personality factors rather than by the pain itself.

Environmental stresses or threatening life-events are more

likely prior to the onset of functional abdominal pain than during a similar period in individuals without pain or in individuals whose pain is due to organic gastrointestinal disease. Clinic visits by IBS patients may be precipitated by a death in the family (cancer), a marriage breakup, or the loss of a job. There have been 2 studies of the emotional state of patients undergoing appendectomy for acute abdominal pain. Compared to those patients with a diseased appendix, individuals with a normal appendix were more likely to have suffered a serious life-event, to be female, to have psychological symptoms or depression, and to suffer persistent gut complaints.

Psychiatrists and psychologists describe learned illness or learned pain behavior. Perhaps, as children, some patients are rewarded for being ill with sympathy or by avoidance of unpleasant activities. We should recall William Whitehead's observation that subjects with a painful irritable bowel were more likely than peptic ulcer sufferers, or those with no pain, to have multiple somatic complaints, to view their colds as more serious than those of other people, and to consult a physician for minor illnesses. They also tended to have received gifts and special food when ill as children. Germane to this observation is the tendency of recurrent abdominal pain in childhood to persist into adult life, and the probability that individuals with nonorganic abdominal pain have had parents who suffered abdominal pain.

In his classic paper "Psychogenic Pain and the Pain-Prone Patient," Engel stated that guilt is an invariable factor in the choice of pain as a symptom. Personality features include masochism, abuse as a child, onset when things were going well, and life-long continued pain and suffering. Engel claimed that "the relish with which the pain-prone patient recounts his tale of suffering alerts the physician that such is an unconscious source of gratification" (1959). No doubt such a process is at work in the introspective, hypochondriacal, self-important craving for sympathy described by Hutcheson in "abdominal" women. Although no physiological research has been done in this area, it seems unlikely that such patients have a primary motility disorder as the basis of their pain. Some individuals may be hypochondriacal, convinced that they have a disease, and fearing the disease, become preoccupied with their bodies. Some may have hysteria or somatization disorder (Chapter 7), whereas many others are simply depressed.

Factitious Pain

Some complainers of abdominal pain are malingering. Often there is an obvious secondary gain, perhaps dependent upon the outcome of a disability ruling or a damage suit. Here physician, patient, and insurer are in a bind, because the pain will not resolve until the legal issue is settled, and the patient's continued complaints can only delay the settlement.

More obscure is the Münchhausen syndrome. The bizarre medical and personal history related by the Münchhausen patient is somehow plausible in the context of a bustling emergency ward, and the attending physician naturally gives him or her the benefit of the doubt. Such patients submit themselves to an awesome array of costly and dangerous procedures, including surgery. Once the "game is up," a Münchhausen usually signs out of hospital and moves on to another center, leaving the physician perplexed. No coherent physiologic or psychologic mechanism has been forthcoming, and there is no satisfactory treatment.

DIAGNOSIS

Say ye, oppress'd by some fantastic woes,
Some jarring nerve that baffles your repose;
. . . Who with sad prayers the weary doctor tease,
To name the nameless ever new disease.

George Crabbe (1754–1832), "The Village"

It goes without saying that the physician should be alert to the possibility that chronic recurrent abdominal pain might be due to organic illness. Cholelithiasis, cholecystitis, peptic ulcer, neph-

rolithiasis, pyelonephritis, Crohn's disease, diverticulitis, and sub-
acute bowel obstruction may produce episodes of pain over many
months or years. Attention to the details of history and physical
examination and notation of fever, weight loss, melena, anemia,
or an elevation of the erythrocyte sedimentation rate should alert
the physician to a structural medical or surgical disorder. Often
patients with the chronic abdomen will have symptoms resembling
one or two of these illnesses and require their exclusion.

The greatest difficulty in the diagnosis of the chronic abdomen
is uncertainty, which engenders insecurity in the physician. Without the conviction of a positive diagnosis, the physician carries little
credibility with the patient, who is usually seeking a ready answer.
To begin, the physician should attempt to relate pain temporally
and anatomically with body function. Epigastric pain, which is
associated with eating, occurs at night, and is relieved by antacids,
suggests a peptic ulcer. Abdominal tenderness is no guide, since
it is equally prevalent in ulcer and nonulcer dyspepsia. Endoscopy
will best settle these issues, and those individuals with no ulcer
may be said to have nonulcer dyspepsia (Chapter 11).

There are now data establishing that a positive diagnosis of
the IBS can be made with a high degree of accuracy. As discussed
in the previous chapter, the IBS can be recognized by a relationship
of the abdominal pain to defecation and by accompanying bowel
symptoms (see Table 13). A diagnosis of the irritable bowel made
by an experienced physician needs no change over time, provided
no new symptoms intervene (see Table 14).

At this point, special mention should be made of biliary colic.
In fact, biliary tract pain is rarely colicky. Recurrent, often nocturnal
attacks of steady epigastric or right upper quadrant abdominal
pain, lasting for 15 minutes or for 1 to 2 days, point to stones in
the biliary tree. An ultrasound examination is necessary to detect
gallstones (see Chapter 22). If none are found and if the pain is
unrelated to meals or bowel habit, it may not be possible to make
a diagnosis. Some individuals may have "biliary dyskinesia," and
sphincter of Oddi spasm may be suspected if there is a transient
rise in the blood of liver enzymes or of bilirubin during an attack.
Note again, however, that such pain may be reproduced in indi-

viduals by intraluminal balloon distension of the upper gut. Pressure measurement of the bile ducts is an infant science, and biliarylike pain should not be attributed to biliary dysfunction without objective evidence, such as accompanying liver test abnormalities in the blood, or stones or dilated ducts upon ultrasound examination.

Other Chronic Pain Syndromes

In those individuals whose pain is unrelated to bodily function, a precise functional diagnosis is impossible. Frequently, the pain is continuous and may radiate beyond the abdomen. Sometimes it is vague and moves from place to place. In others, it is described with "relish" in colorful detail. The physician should look for a secondary gain (eg, a financial or social need to be ill), recent stressful events, and, most importantly, symptoms of depression. The only physical signs are the facial expression of depression and the abdominal scars resulting from fruitless surgery to which such patients are prone. Hysteria, pain-proneness, and the use of narcotics are more likely in individuals who have had multiple surgery.

Because patients with the chronic abdomen may have a psychological or personality disorder, it may be anxiety or depression that brings them to the doctor. In those bizarre or persistent pains that make little physiologic sense, the psychiatric condition may be an integral part or cause of the pain. There is still a stigma attached to mental symptoms, and many people consider them an indication of personal failure. It is still unacceptable for some people to regard themselves as emotionally ill. Thus, psychiatric illness may have to assume a physical guise. Therefore, the physician must be alert to the presence of depression, hypochondriasis (the need of the illness to cover personal failure), hysteria (symbolic disability), pain proneness (masochism to atone for guilt), and paranoid schizophrenia. For the schizophrenic patient, a psychiatrist is necessary, but other patients can usually be managed by the physician.

MANAGEMENT

We see too many scarred abdomens with persistence of symptoms, too many "re-operations" and operations undertaken for pain.

J. A. Ryle (1928)

Those who are caring for or who are suffering with the chronic abdomen must be mindful of William Osler's dictum to do no harm. As defined here, the chronic abdomen is a benign disease in a physical sense, but invasive tests and even surgery can cause real morbidity and undermine confidence in the diagnosis. Based on a diagnosis that confidently excludes organic disease, therefore, the physician should develop a strategy of management that includes sympathetic exploration of psychosocial factors, explanation and reassurance, minimal use of drugs and tests, and a follow-up plan that is designed to provide continued support (see Chapter 13). Most physicians suspect the chronic abdomen on the first or second visit. They may identify one of the symptom patterns, such as the irritable bowel syndrome, or be impressed by features that do not follow any pathologic pattern. The necessary diagnostic tests should be done in the first instance to reassure both patient and physician and to avoid the necessity of having them done later in a way that further weakens confidence in the diagnosis.

Time spent discussing the patient's problems and attempting to explain how his or her symptoms can occur without any structural disease should pay dividends later. It is the insistence by some patients with the chronic abdomen that there *must* be something wrong and hitherto overlooked that makes the pain so difficult to manage.

Individuals with the irritable bowel, particularly if they are constipated, may notice some improvement in bowel function with the use of bran. This procedure helps build up their confidence, even though it might not help the pain very much. Similarly, in nonulcer dyspepsia, many patients benefit from a placebo response to antacids, even though there is no rationale of their use. Certainly, bran or small-dose antacids are preferable to systemic drugs.

Table 21
Psychiatric or Personality Disorders Associated with the Chronic
Abdomen[a]

Psychiatric entity	Management
Depression or depressive equivalent	Tricyclic antidepressants
Hypochondriasis	Regular brief visits (placebo)
Conversion/hysteria	Follow-up visits and family therapy
Pain-prone (masochism)	Minimize tests, drugs
	Management of guilt feelings
Somatic delusions (paranoid schizophrenia)	Psychiatric referral

[a] Reproduced with permission from the *Hospital Physician* (1971;6:68–72).

A small, blinded preliminary study reported that sphincter-otomy (incision of the SO) over a 4-year period improved the pain in patients with motor abnormalities of the bile ducts. However, experience is necessary before this hazardous procedure can be recommended for regular use. It is likely that most biliary-type pain in the absence of gallstones is not biliary dyskinesia.

In patients with functional abdominal pain, especially if no associated gut symptoms exist, the physician should look for psychiatric or personality disorders. The disorders that are commonly found include depression, hypochondriasis, hysteria, pain-prone-ness, and paranoid schizophrenia (Table 21).

The *depressed* patient may benefit from a tricyclic antidepressant drug, even if the depression is not obvious. If the patient reports no improvement after several weeks or if there is a threat of suicide, the physician should consider psychiatric referral.

The *hypochondriac* has a sense of personal failure or inadequacy. Unable to admit this to himself, he unconsciously presents as physically rather than psychologically impaired. Telling a hypochondriac that he obviously is not sick is of no avail. He needs to be in someone's care and is often satisfied by regular brief appointments several weeks apart. Inert placebos with no side effects help demonstrate this care until the patient trusts the doctor enough to discuss his problems of living.

Hysterical patients have abdominal pain or other disability for more complex reasons. The pain, which may carry great symbolic meaning, may require psychiatric methods to unravel. The physician can try to help the patient to deal with the conflicts that he or she encounters in life. Family involvement also seems important.

Hutcheson described assumption of the *pain-prone* patient's care as a "bleak prospect," and suggested the need for "something which will dislocate the patient's mind from its perpetual revolution around her umbilicus and set it open to wider horizons." Engel observed that such patients are worse when things are going well for them, yet their histories are a litany of painful illnesses and injuries with redundant tests and therapies, often including surgery. It is as if some personal disaster serves to assuage their guilt. A psychiatric consultation may be helpful, but it is usually the physician who must provide ongoing care. In the individual with learned illness behavior, the physician needs to stop the reward for being sick. This usually involves the complicity of friends or relatives.

Pain-prone patients are often highly critical of their previous physicians. Some suffer so vividly and cry out for relief of pain so plaintively that they "stir rescue fantasies in the most case-hardened doctor." As succinctly put by Tryer,

> to attempt to change the habits of a life time—particularly if these remain advantageous to the patient and his family—may prove an unreasonable contract; the therapist is entitled to retire to the wings if no progress is possible.

Notwithstanding, the physician and the family, however limited the goals might be, must continue to support the patient and at least defend him from illness due to the complications of tests or drugs.

In many cases, cure is an unrealistic goal. The physician should try to help the patient cope with stress and offer continued concern and care.

> To cure sometimes, to relieve often, to comfort always.
>
> Anonymous

SUMMARY

Chronic abdominal pain is common and includes several syndromes and pseudosyndromes. Recurrent attacks of organic disease, such as peptic ulcer or biliary colic, can be identified by a careful history, whereas most of the remaining cases will reveal no pathology. The physician should attempt to identify and treat such syndromes as the irritable bowel or functional dyspepsia. Those patients who have pain with no connection to gastrointestinal function, or even those patients with the irritable bowel who fail to improve with the usual measures, may be suffering from depression, hypochondriasis, hysteria, pain-proneness, or schizophrenia. The latter requires psychiatric consultation. The other psychological problems, however, must be managed by the physician, who, along with the patient, may find the exercise frustrating. A positive diagnosis of functional abdominal pain is essential in order to avoid unnecessary tests and drugs. Some patients may respond to a reassurance that no serious disease exists, but most may require continuing care, with repeated visits that will reassure them, help them to cope with stressful situations, and attempt to modify their illness behavior.

Once a careful physical assessment has been done and the appropriate tests are completed, the patient with the chronic abdomen must be persuaded that additional consultation is futile and that further tests and drug treatments may be a greater threat to health than the pain itself. The lingering suspicion in the mind of the patient that the physician has missed something, or that there is a cure which everyone has overlooked, is the great enemy of sensible management.

CHAPTER FIFTEEN

Functional Diarrhea

Diarrhea is an important component of the irritable bowel syndrome (IBS). When accompanied with abdominal pain, alternating constipation, and the other features of the IBS that are discussed in Chapter 13, the diagnosis is not difficult. However, when the diarrhea occurs alone or as the dominant feature, special problems arise. In this chapter it is pertinent to discuss the definition of functional diarrhea, its possible mechanisms, its differentiation from some of the common organic causes of chronic diarrhea, and its management.

DEFINITION

As was discussed in Chapter 3, no universally accepted definition of diarrhea exists. An ideal description would consider frequency, consistency, effort/urgency, and intestinal or whole gut transit time. For the reasons that were discussed in that chapter, transit time is of little clinical value. Many studies consider more than 3 movements a day as diarrhea, but this would include some individuals with formed or pelletlike stools. Furthermore, the diarrhea may be intermittent. Instead, we have adopted the operational definition of "loose or watery stools on more than 75 percent of occasions" as being most likely to satisfy the need to include all individuals with significant diarrhea and to exclude those who have several normal or constipated stools daily.

Because there are many known causes of chronic diarrhea, a positive diagnosis by history of functional diarrhea is less easy than that of most gut reactions. In some patients, extensive testing is necessary to exclude organic disease. Furthermore, new causes of diarrhea are being recognized over time, such as lactose intolerance, bile salt malabsorption, and inadvertent sorbitol ingestion. However, a substantial number of people present with chronic, sometimes painless, persistent or recurrent diarrhea which the physician may readily identify, from a careful history, as functional.

One final point. There are a myriad of toxins, viruses, bacteria, medications, and environmental circumstances that may cause a self-limiting diarrhea. Unless the sufferer is very ill, diagnosis is often not made, and with patience the episode passes. We are concerned in this chapter only with chronic diarrhea. Thus, functional diarrhea may be defined as a functional disorder of at least 3 months' duration consisting of loose, watery stools on more than 75 percent of occasions.

MECHANISMS OF DIARRHEA

Normal defecation depends upon normal function of the small intestine, colon, rectum, and anal sphincters. We have seen in Chapter 2 that the small gut daily handles about 8 liters of fluid containing nutrients and minerals from diet and secretions and presents about 1 liter of this fluid to the colon. The colon absorbs most of this fluid and has a finite reserve absorption capacity. Intricately intertwined with these fluid shifts are the peristaltic activity of the small intestine and the mixing and segmenting activity of the colon. The rectum stores up to 200 grams of stool before defecation is triggered, and the anal sphincter prevents leaking or inadvertent evacuation.

Disturbances of any of these components can result in diarrhea. For example, the rapid small-bowel transit seen in hyper-thyroidism allows for insufficient absorption of fluid and nutrients and delivers a load to the colon beyond its capacity to salvage the overflow. Celiac disease, which may impair small gut mucosal ab-sorption of glucose and other small molecules, or chronic pan-creatitis, which impairs digestion of large protein, fat, or carbo-hydrate molecules, results in the retention of osmotically active molecules in the gut lumen. The hyperosmotic gut contents then attract water into the gut, again overwhelming the colon. Osmotic laxatives, such as lactulose or milk of magnesia, act in a similar manner (see Chapter 19).

Certain diseases induce a "secretory diarrhea" in which the small gut is induced to secrete (or not absorb) water. Bacterial tox-ins, such as those of cholera or toxigenic *Escherichia coli*, the cause of traveler's diarrhea, act in this way as do the "stimulant laxa-tives." Extremely rare chronic secretory diarrheas occur with islet cell tumors of the pancreas or medullary carcinoma of the thyroid. Unlike osmotic diarrhea, secretory diarrhea continues during fast-ing.

Following vagotomy, cholecystectomy, or removal of the ileum, increased bile salts may reach the colon. Bile salts stimulate colon secretion and motility thus causing diarrhea. The colon's ability to absorb even a normal small gut residue may be impaired by inflammation of the mucosa, such as occurs with colitis. An inflamed colon mucosal surface may exude fluid into the lumen. As observed previously, decreased contraction of the colon may fail to brake the fecal flow. An inflamed or irritable rectum may not tolerate a normal stool volume and may prematurely signal defecation. Many antibiotics cause diarrhea, presumably by killing some bacteria and allowing others to survive. Finally, in some diar-rhea patients who are bothered by incontinence, the anal sphincter is found to be weak.

Whatever the cause of the diarrhea, it is rare to find only one of the above mechanisms at work. The defect in functional diarrhea is unknown, although some studies identify rapid transit, in-creased small-bowel residue, decreased colon contractions, or re-duced sphincter pressure. It is possible that there are many causes, or that the enteric nervous system malfunctions (perhaps influenced by the emotions) and produces gut incoordination involving several of the above mechanisms.

DIAGNOSIS

History

The first step in diagnosis is to determine if the patient indeed has diarrhea. Upon questioning, many patients reveal that they are passing frequent, hard, round, or narrow pieces, which are often described as rabbit stools or sheep stools (depending, I suppose, on one's barnyard experience). Doctors call such stools *scybala*. (I know a physician who uses photographs to help patients identify their stool type, but have never brought myself to follow his example.) A typical IBS patient will describe hard stools in the morning followed shortly by 2 or 3 progressively looser ones. Other patients may be constipated for long periods and are relieved only by a burst of hard and then loose stools. In these cases, it is doubtful if diagnosis needs further pursuit.

The second step is to decide whether the diarrhea is most likely functional, requiring a minimal inquiry, or organic, requiring a more extensive investigation. There are a number of clues that may help in the decision (Table 22). In Western clinics, the functional patient will likely be well nourished, female, and between 15 and 60 years of age. The diarrhea, which may have been present for many years, is often intermittent, and may alternate with constipation or normal movements. Like the IBS, it may date from a stressful life-event, the use of a drug, or from an attack of gastroenteritis. Scybala, mucus, feeling of distension, and lack of satisfaction after defecation are characteristics of the IBS. If abdominal pain is present, it is relieved by defecation and may herald a change in stool frequency or consistency. None of these features are diagnostic, however, but the more that are present, the more likely the patient has the IBS or functional diarrhea (see Chapter 13). The physician should also take care to ask about incontinence, which

Table 22
Historic Features That Help to Distinguish Functional and Organic Types of Chronic Diarrhea[a]

Feature	Functional	Organic
Female (in Western clinics)	+	—
Well-nourished	+	—
Long-standing diarrhea	+	—
Emotional instability or stress	+	—
Onset with gastroenteritis, bereavement, or cathartics	+	—
Intermittent or alternating with constipation	+	—
Mucus	+	—
Scybala	+	—
Abdominal distension	+	—
Pain relief with defecation	+	—
Pain heralds onset of diarrhea	+	—
Morning diarrhea	+	—
Continuous, watery stools	—	+
Nocturnal diarrhea	—	+
Weight loss	—	+
<15 years or >60 years (onset)	—	+
Fever	—	+
Blood in stool	—	+
Anemia	—	+
Pus in stool	—	+
Greasy, foul, floating stools	—	+
>5 movements/day	—	+
Incontinence	±	+
Previous gastrointestinal surgery	—	+

[a] Adapted from Thompson WG: *The Irritable Gut*. Baltimore, University Park Press, 1979, p. 86.

can occur with any diarrhea and may be the most troublesome aspect to the sufferer.

On the other hand, if diarrhea is accompanied by pus or blood in the stool, or if there is fever, weight loss, anemia, loss of appetite, or vomiting, the explanation is not functional. Nocturnal diarrhea or more than 4 or 5 loose stools per day is more likely to occur in organic disease. Previous gastrointestinal surgery may indicate a structural cause for the diarrhea. It is unknown whether emotional problems are more common in functional than in organic diarrhea, but an individual who chronically passes many loose stools is likely to be anxious or depressed on that account.

It is important to stress that the functional and organic categories are not mutually exclusive. A patient with functional diarrhea is not immune to organic conditions, such as celiac disease or regional enteritis. A good history, therefore, is vital. Examination should detect systemic illnesses, such as hyperthyroidism, that could account for the diarrhea.

The history should also include a detailed survey of the diarrhea sufferer's habits, drug use, and dietary practices in relation to the diarrhea. Alcohol abuse can cause diarrhea, and many individuals have a problem with red wine or beer. Gum chewers should take care that the gum does not include sorbitol, mannitol, or fructose, since these artificial sweeteners are also laxatives. In some, the diarrhea disappears when the sufferer stops gum, candies, or soft drinks containing artificial sweeteners. Many drugs cause diarrhea. It is surprising how many sufferers are habitually using laxatives or other medications which they do not relate to their diarrhea (see Chapters 19 and 20). Most antacids contain milk of magnesia, which is a laxative. Antibiotics, too, and some cardiac drugs are suspect. The history of diarrhea, cramps, and gas after milk ingestion, especially in non-Caucasians, should suggest lactose intolerance. Campers and travelers to endemic areas may have acquired the *Giardia* parasite.

Much is made in the lay press of food allergies. Certainly, some individuals get a bowel upset and "hives" from shellfish or strawberries, but, in general, allergy is a rare cause of diarrhea alone. Pursuit of the notion that it is something in the diet seldom leads to a viable diagnosis or a lasting cure.

Investigation

Any patient with diarrhea should, after careful history and physical examination, have blood drawn for hemoglobin estima-

Table 23
Common Causes of Chronic Diarrhea That
Might Mistakenly Be Called Functional

Ingested substances
  Alcohol
  Excessive coffee or tea
  Sorbitol, mannitol, fructose
  Milk (in lactose-intolerant people)
  Laxative abuse (overt or surreptitious)
  Drugs
Systemic disease
  Hyperthyroidism
Infection
  Giardia lamblia
Malassimilation of diet
  Celiac disease—impaired mucosal absorption
  Chronic pancreatitis—impaired digestion
Inflammatory bowel disease
  Crohn's disease
  Ulcerative colitis
Villous adenoma

tion, white cell count, and a sedimentation rate estimation. A sigmoidoscopic examination is important as well (Chapter 22). Fresh stool may be obtained for culture and search for ova and parasites. If the patient is over 40, it is good medical practice to order a barium enema. If any of these tests suggest organic disease, appropriate investigation should proceed from there.

There are a great many causes of chronic diarrhea, and a complete discussion is not possible here. However, there are several common disorders that should not be missed, and their detection will be discussed briefly (Table 23). In cases in which the degree of diarrhea is doubtful, a 72-hour stool collection may be helpful. Daily output of more than 300 grams of stool on a Western high-fat diet should make the physician think of an organic cause of the disease. The specimen can be analyzed for fat and if that is increased, a malabsorption state, such as celiac disease or maldigestion due to pancreatic disease, is likely. Sometimes a laxative may be discovered in the specimen (Chapter 19). Certainly, a high output or increased stool fat (steatorrhea) demands further investigation. Inflammatory bowel disease of the colon, that is ulcerative colitis or Crohn's colitis, are usually accompanied by blood and pus in the stool, fever, and weight loss. Most cases are diagnosed by sigmoidoscopy. Crohn's disease of the right colon or small bowel may be more difficult, but should be suspected in a young person who has chronic diarrhea, weight loss, fever, or abdominal pain, especially if there is a mass or exquisite tenderness in the right lower quadrant of the abdomen. A small-bowel enema may be necessary to exclude this increasingly common disease (Chapter 22).

As mentioned, few infections cause chronic diarrhea. One that does and is often overlooked is that caused by *Giardia lamblia*, a monocellular parasite that clings to the duodenal mucosa causing a crampy, watery diarrhea with weight loss, fever, and malaise. It is so common in some areas, such as in the Canadian Rockies, that physicians treat patients on the basis of history alone with the antibiotic metronidazole (Flagyl). Because the parasite is carried by beavers and other animals, humans often acquire it by drinking lake water, prompting Westerners to call it "beaver fever." Three separate fresh stool specimens sent to a good bacteriology laboratory will result in identification of the parasite in about 50 percent of cases. Duodenal aspiration or biopsy through a gastroscope is much more reliable. In suspected cases in an endemic area, a trial of therapy with metronidazole seems reasonable.

With one exception, benign and malignant tumors of the gut do not cause chronic diarrhea. That exception is a villous adenoma of the colon or rectum. This tumor consists of long, fernlike processes called *villi*, which exude water, protein, and minerals and may occasionally bleed. If near the lower end of the colon, where reabsorption cannot take place, a mucousy diarrhea results, which is often ignored for months or years. It has great malignant potential and is therefore a very good reason why sigmoidoscopy should be done in individuals who suffer chronic diarrhea.

Thus, the essential investigations for chronic diarrhea should include a careful, complete history, an examination for abdominal masses, detection of signs of nutritional deficiency or anemia, a sigmoidoscopy, and, in the over-40 patient, a barium enema. Further testing depends upon positive findings in the above tests and upon local conditions, but should employ economy and common sense. In the end, most patients with chronic diarrhea who are seen by a primary care physician prove not to have an organic cause.

TREATMENT

The treatment plan for chronic diarrhea should follow that outlined in Chapter 13. The discussion here will concentrate on dietary measures and antidiarrhea drugs.

Dietary Measures

Eat what you want and let the food fight it out inside

Mark Twain (1835–1910)

Obviously, the physician should act on the information of chronic diarrhea gleaned in diagnosis. Gum chewers, alcohol imbibers, and laxative users should modify their habits. If a drug seems a likely cause, a substitute should be found, or a "drug holiday" should be tried. In some individuals with a history suggestive of milk intolerance, a lactose-free diet should be given a 2- to 4-week trial. To be sure, there are tests for lactose intolerance (Chapter 22), but the best one is withdrawal of milk. The lactase enzyme (LactAid) may be added to the milk of lactose-intolerant subjects who need calcium.

The diarrhea of the IBS will often respond to a high-bulk diet employing bran or psyllium, which is a cheap, safe, first maneuver in functional diarrhea. The patient needs to recall that bran is not a laxative in the usual sense but that it may solidify liquid stool and improve gut function generally. If effective, a bulking agent is the best solution to a vexing, benign disorder which may last a lifetime. Therefore, 1 tablespoonful of bran, three times daily, should be given on a 2- to 3-month trial.

Table 24
Antidiarrhea Medications

I. Agents that act in the gut lumen
  A. Dietary fiber
    1. Bran
    2. Psyllium (ispaghula)
    3. Pectin
    4. Agar
  B. Cholestyramine
  C. Aluminum
    1. Kaolin
    2. Aluminum hydroxide
  D. Bismuth
II. Opiate drugs that act on the mucosa, gut wall, or nerve supply
  A. Natural
    1. Morphine
    2. Paregoric (camphorated tincture of opium)
    3. Codeine
  B. Synthetic
    1. Diphenoxylate
    2. Loperamide

Drugs

Cholestyramine

Patients with resection of the ileum, a previous vagotomy, or gallbladder removal may spill bile salts into the colon where they exert a laxative effect (Table 24). Small doses of cholestyramine (Questran) may cause a dramatic improvement. A small number of patients without previous surgery also respond to this drug, so a trial of therapy is reasonable in individuals with chronic, persistent, unexplained diarrhea who do not respond to bran.

Cholestyramine tastes like plastic, which of course it is, and patients taking 30 or more grams per day for high blood cholesterol find it objectionable. Consumption can also risk malabsorption of the fat-soluble vitamins A, D, K, and E. Only 4 to 6 grams of cholestyramine are necessary to treat bile-salt diarrhea, and, at this dose, the taste and vitamin malabsorption are less troublesome. It is the grittiness of the bile-salt binding resin that is unpleasant. If the patient can be bothered to do so, 0.5 grams of the powder may be placed in a gelatin capsule. Alternatively, the drug may be disguised with meals in a variety of ways. For this purpose, it may be added to concentrated orange juice, mayonnaise on a celery stick, peanut butter, or a cheese sauce. If the drug works, the sufferer will need no persuasion to continue it. Unlike the treatment of hypercholesterolemia, the results of cholestyramine in bile-salt wasting diarrhea are obvious and immediate. For example:

> a 70 year old woman with diarrhea that began suddenly 14 years previously produced up to 10 watery movements daily and in the last decade diarrhea was continuous. She lost no weight but was socially incapacitated. Physical examination, sigmoidscopy and barium enema were negative. Lactose tolerance test and 3 day stool fat estimation were also normal. Bran, diphenoxylate, and codeine were of little benefit. Within a few days of commencing cholestyramine she began passing her first formed movements in 10 years.

Aluminum

Kaolin, which is a hydrated aluminum citrate, is a time-honored remedy for diarrhea and is believed to bind bacteria, toxins, and other substances. Aluminum hydroxide also has a constipating effect, which accounts for its addition to antacid mixtures containing milk of magnesia. Even though no one knows how it works, aluminum hydroxide does bind bile acids. There has been little study of the efficacy of these intraluminally acting substances in the treatment of functional diarrhea.

Pectin

Pectin from citrus rind is hydrophilic and is classed as a dietary fiber (Chapter 6). For many years, it has been used in antidiarrheal mixtures especially in combination with kaolin. Because pectin is almost totally destroyed in the gut, its mode of action, if there is any, is a mystery.

Bismuth

For many years, bismuth subsalicylate has been marketed for the treatment of diarrhea and dyspepsia under the trade name Pepto-Bismol. Ignored until recently by pharmacologists, this substance is effective in the treatment of traveler's diarrhea, a self-limited disorder that is due to bacterial toxins acquired in tropical countries. There is interest in the possible use of bismuth in the treatment of chronic gastritis, which may be caused by the newly recognized organism *Helicobacter pylori* (Chapter 11). Bismuth subsalicylate reduces subjective complaints of diarrhea, nausea, and the abdominal cramping caused by the toxins of *E. coli* and *Shigella*. The compound is thought to have a specific action against enteric bacterial toxins. If this is true, it would not be expected to be useful in functional diarrhea. Users should not be alarmed to discover that, like iron, bismuth may blacken the stools.

Anticholinergics

As discussed in Chapter 13, when given in doses that cause side effects, anticholinergics reduce segmental contractions, which, however, might be expected to make diarrhea worse. In any case, their benefit is still unproven (see Chapter 21).

Opiates

The opiates are a group of alkaloids that are derived from opium, of which *morphine* is the prototype. Their mechanism of action will be treated in Chapter 20. Their antidiarrheal effect is believed to be due to increased colon segmental contractions, prolonged transit, and perhaps increased net water absorption in the small bowel. Constipation is a well-known side effect of morphine and codeine, and, until recently, paregoric (camphorated tincture of opium) was used at "subanalgesic" dosages as a popular antidiarrheal preparation. Over short periods, paregoric is quite effective, but its addictive potential and the availability of safer, newer drugs has made it obsolete. *Codeine* is less addictive and expensive, and if prescribed at a dose of 30 milligrams 2 or 3 times daily, is superior to anticholinergics in the treatment of diarrhea. However, it does have an effect on the central nervous system, which makes it unsatisfactory for chronic diarrhea.

Diphenoxylate (Lomotil) is a synthetic opiate with less addicting potential which, in a 2.5-milligram dose, is as effective as 4 milliliters of paregoric in controlling diarrhea. The maximum dose is 5 tablets per day. Because the drug has some addicting potential, it requires a prescription in many jurisdictions.

Loperamide (Imodium) is said to have no central nervous system effects and requires no prescription. It is more potent than diphenoxylate and longer acting. The usefulness of loperamide in acute diarrhea is undoubted, but there are few good studies of its employment in chronic functional diarrhea. Unlike diphenoxylate, it increases anal sphincter tone and, therefore, may be of some benefit in patients who have incontinence associated with their diarrhea. One 2-milligram tablet is recommended following each loose bowel movement up to a maximum of 8 tablets per day. However, this dose may be too much for chronic diarrhea.

If bulking agents and avoidance of provoking factors fail to control functional diarrhea, the physician may consider use of a drug, and loperamide appears to be the best choice. But if the diarrhea is chronic, continued use is unwise unless the diarrhea is disabling. In the IBS, overuse of an opiate in the diarrheal phase may aggravate the constipated phase, escalating the intestinal dysfunction. One strategy is to use the drug only before important or stressful engagements during which an urgent trip to the toilet would be a social or professional embarrassment.

SUMMARY

Functional diarrhea is a functional disorder of at least 3 months' duration that typically consists of loose or watery stools on more than 75 percent of occasions. In gastroenterology clinics, the disorder is commonly seen in well-nourished females and frequently accompanies emotional instability. The cause is unknown but likely involves altered secretion and motility of the small bowel, colon, and rectum. Incontinence that is due to an apparently weakened anal sphincter distresses some individuals. It can often begin with gastroenteritis, a bereavement, or cathartic abuse. Scybala, distension, mucus, alternation with constipation, and other features discussed in Chapter 13 suggest the irritable bowel, but it is persistent watery diarrhea that challenges the physician's diagnostic acumen. Diarrhea sufferers should also be aware that lactose may cause diarrhea and that some artificial sweeteners are also laxatives. Weight loss, fever, nocturnal diarrhea, more than 5 movements per day, recent onset, and extremes of age suggest an organic cause. The passage of blood, pus, or foul, greasy, floating movements demands investigation. Table 23 lists common organic causes from which functional diarrhea is usually distinguished by a careful history, physical examination, and sigmoidoscopy. In all cases, the patient's psychosocial situation should be discussed sympathetically, the benign character of the disorder explained, and follow-up assured. Therapy should be aimed first at mopping up the stool with such bulking agents as bran or psyllium. Occasionally, cholestyramine may be beneficial. If a drug is necessary because of disability, the safest and most effective is loperamide, although codeine and diphenoxylate still enjoy wide popularity. If possible, use of these agents should be restricted to periods of increased disability or prior to important engagements.

CHAPTER SIXTEEN

Constipation

The concept of regularity is one of the most enduring myths that has been handed down to us by our forefathers. Since antiquity, an empty colon has been equated with purity; and what generations of mothers have believed, let no one belittle. Nevertheless, daily elimination is not essential to health, and probably occurs in only about one half of adults. As discussed in Chapter 3, normal people have between 3 movements per week and 3 per day. Even the 1 percent of individuals who fall outside this range are not necessarily abnormal. In 1813, the British physician Heberdon described a patient who "never went but once a month." The world's record for rectal continence is held by a man who resisted the temptations of the toilet for 368 days. "There was much rejoicing in the family" on June 21, 1901, when he delivered 36 liters of feces. By anyone's definition, this is constipation, but the exact limits of normal bowel habits remain unclear. In most cases, the frequency of defecation is less important than the consistency of the stool, the effort necessary to expel it, and the associated symptoms.

TYPES OF CONSTIPATION

Constipation may be functional or organic. As we come to understand the functional causes better, undoubtedly they will be

Table 25
Types of Constipation

A. Functional
   1. Irritable bowel
   2. Colonic inertia (pseudo-obstruction)
   3. Spastic pelvic floor/anismus
   4. Megacolon
   5. Denied bowel motion syndrome
B. Organic
   1. Obstructive—cancer, stricture
   2. Retentive—fissure in ano, proctitis
   3. Metabolic—hypothyroidism
   4. Pharmacologic—opiates, phenothiazines, tranquilizers, tricyclic antidepressants, calcium channel blockers, bismuth, iron, calcium, aluminum
   5. Neurogenic—spinal cord injury, brain damage, enteric nerve damage or loss (Hirschsprung's disease, pseudo-obstruction)
   6. Muscle damage—pseudo-obstruction, scleroderma
   7. Depression

added to the organic list Table 25. Classification of the functional causes of constipation is difficult. Although certain motor or sensory abnormalities have been identified, they are not sufficiently precise to label them organic. There is much overlap among these functional syndromes, and pharmacologic and surgical attempts to correct the putative motor abnormalities have not been very successful.

Functional Constipation

Irritable Bowel Syndrome (IBS)

As discussed in Chapter 13, the constipation of the IBS is accompanied by abdominal pain that is relieved by defecation. The stools, which are characteristically hard, often like sheep stools (scybala), are passed with much straining. The trauma of their passage may result in anal fissures or bleeding hemorrhoids. Also there may be intervals of diarrhea. The colon is sensitive to dis-

tension, and many researchers believe that increased colon segmental contraction holds back the stool and compresses it, so that
the rectum is often empty or contains only a few small, hard scybala. Simulated stools placed in the rectum demonstrate that the
smaller the stool, the more difficult it is to expel. It has been estimated that at least 200 grams of stool are necessary to adequately
stimulate the defecation reflex. The 130-gram stool commonly
found in Western societies does not measure up.

The role of fiber deficiency and emotion in the IBS is discussed
in Chapter 13. The constipation of the IBS is the feature most likely
to respond to a high-fiber diet. Stool output has been noted to be
less in introverted individuals who describe themselves in unfa-
vorable terms. Thus, good results may be expected from a high-
fiber diet and attention to psychological difficulties.

Colon Inertia

In some constipated patients, normal contractions are reduced, and colonic transit is prolonged. Sir Arthur Hurst, the pioneering British physiologist, called failure of the rectum to contract *dyschezia*. In extreme cases there may be smooth muscle or
enteric ganglia degeneration in the colon. Called *chronic intestinal
pseudo-obstruction*, this is a recently recognized organic disorder
often occurring in families. Pseudo-obstruction may present with
symptoms and signs that mimic mechanical obstruction of the
colon, and sometimes surgery is needed to exclude that possibility.
Removal of the colon is usually unsuccessful treatment. Since the
entire gut is affected by this disorder, obstruction may occur elsewhere postoperatively. Pseudo-obstruction patients have widespread dysfunction of smooth muscle resulting in such divergent
symptoms as difficulty in swallowing, sterility, miscarriage, incomplete bladder emptying, and so on.

Intestinal pseudo-obstruction should be regarded as an extreme cause of colonic inertia. In most cases, surgery is not performed, and no pathologic findings, if any exist, are discovered.
Colonic inertia other than pseudo-obstruction occurs almost exclusively in women. In this condition, colon transit is delayed and

although the constipation is severe, it is often painless. The laxative bisacodyl (Dulcolax), which stimulates powerful contractions in normal colons, fails to do so in many individuals with inertia. Although psychological disturbances, even psychoses, are reported, they may, like other functional disorders, be cause, effect, or coincidence. Thus, management of colon inertia is extremely difficult and the results of surgery can often be disastrous.

Spastic Pelvic Floor and Anismus

Another cause of severe, fiber-resistant constipation found in young and middle-aged women is that due to failure of the pelvic floor or external anal sphincter to relax during defecation. These women have extremely slow colon transit and are unable to expel simulated stool from the rectum. Normally, during attempts at defecation, the puborectalis muscle relaxes, straightening the sharp anorectal angle (see Figure 8). In these constipated women, this relaxation fails to occur, and the external anal sphincter paradoxically may tighten during straining. These observations explain why laxatives and removal of the colon above the rectum fail to improve the constipation.

Similar phenomena are observed when the parasympathetic nerve supply to the distal colon has been damaged, suggesting a neurologic cause for the discoordinated pelvic floor. It might also explain why many women with colonic inertia date the onset of their constipation to childbirth or hysterectomy, during which damage to the pelvic nerves might have occurred. In most cases, however, the constipation commences in childhood or adolescence and worsens over the next 20 years. One study suggested a genetic cause for the spastic pelvic floor based on characteristic fingerprints.

There also appears to be an association of constipation with other pelvic floor abnormalities. Rectal prolapse occurs when bowel is forced through a weakened anal sphincter. This can result in an intense urge to strain which, of course, makes matters worse. Some women whose puborectalis fails to relax seem to force feces against the vagina thereby creating a rectocele (rectum bulge into vagina).

They may succeed in passing stool only when they press backward with their fingers in the vagina. In such cases, surgical repair of the rectocele offers some hope of improvement.

Megacolon/Megarectum

A small number of patients with constipation have a large, dilated rectum or colon that is poorly responsive to rectal distension and laxatives. Frequently, fecal impaction and soiling date from childhood, and many such individuals have urine retention as well. This abnormality may be due to primary damage of the colon nerve supply or it may be secondary to chronic fecal loading. The latter cause may explain its frequency in mentally deficient or psychotic individuals. Occasionally, such patients plug the toilet with a giant evacuation.

It is essential that megacolon be distinguished from treatable colonic lesions, such as an anal stricture, or Hirschsprung's disease (see Organic Constipation). Laxatives are of no avail, and may make matters worse (see Chapter 19).

Denied Bowel Movements

Some people claim to be severely constipated who clearly are not. This condition may be due to a misunderstanding or misperception that can only be clarified by a period of observation in the hospital. In a few cases, however, there appears to be a deliberate attempt to mislead. Such persons deny defecation, even though orally administered radio-opaque markers can be seen through successive abdominal x-rays to disappear from their colon. Münchhausen's syndrome is the term often appended to patients who deliberately provide false, often preposterous histories and then subject themselves to needless, sometimes harmful investigation and treatment, even surgery (Chapter 14).

Organic Constipation

Constipation results from a wide variety of local and systemic disorders, some of which are listed in Table 25. These disorders must be considered before one can make a diagnosis of functional constipation. Perianal conditions, such as fissures or localized proctitis, may lead to conscious or subconscious defense of the area by the withholding of stool. Cancer of the colon or diverticulitis are causes of recent changes in bowel habit in middle-aged people and must be rigorously excluded. In hypothyroidism, replacement of the missing thyroid hormone may be curative. Remember especially that many drugs, including codeine, phenothiazines, calcium channel blockers, beta blockers, and certain heavy metals are constipating (Chapter 20). Brain or spinal cord injury destroys appreciation of the need to defecate, whereas damage to the lower spinal cord or pelvic nerves may interfere with motor function.

Hirschsprung's disease is characterized by an absence of myenteric nerve ganglia in the anal canal and lower rectum. Usually discovered in childhood, the denervated segment fails to function, thus causing obstruction with a dilated colon above. Distension of the rectum fails to relax the internal anal sphincter. Occasionally, the diagnosis is made in adulthood through rectal biopsies showing absence of ganglia.

Depression is a common cause of constipation and the matter is worsened by some drugs that are used to treat it, particularly the tricyclic antidepressants.

FACTORS INFLUENCING CONSTIPATION

Many factors in ourselves, in our habits, and in our environment appear to contribute to constipation. Constipation increases with age. The elderly and the mentally or physically handicapped may ignore calls to stool and retain their feces. Infants may discover that refusal to defecate is an effective strategy to gain parental attention. Sixteen percent of women are constipated just before menstruation and many others are troubled during pregnancy. Sex hormones that delay colon transit in animals may be responsible, but mechanical factors are important also. In some women, constipation dates from childbirth or hysterectomy.

The importance of dietary fiber to normal defecation has been discussed earlier, but fluids are equally important. In Australia, constipation is a summer disease due to dehydration and is corrected simply by extra fluids.

Squatting is thought to be the ideal position for defecation. For this reason, the high toilet seat has been criticized (Chapter 2). It would seem to be particularly disadvantageous to a small child whose legs may dangle unsupported over an adult-sized toilet seat.

Inconvenient toilets are more than a nuisance, because they may force one to retain stool, thus impairing the defecation reflex. Further, shy persons may be self-conscious about going to a public facility. Early in this century, such famous physicians as Sir Arthur Hurst complained of the poorly lit, uncomfortable, and unventilated toilets that discouraged their use. It seems that we have progressed little since that time. Even the most determined supplicant hesitates to enter the filthy, fly-infested service station toilets that pollute our highways or the neglected public toilets in any downtown area.

Inactivity, such as that following surgery or illness, may be costive. Constipation has been blamed on weakness of the abdominal muscles in disabled patients; however, the majority of normal individuals are unaware of straining. Furthermore, a 5-year-old boy with congenital absence of abdominal muscles had no difficulty in defecating, which demonstrates that the gut can "go it alone." Disability is more likely to result in poor appetite, poor nutrition of gut muscles, embarrassment, or an improper position at defecation.

Undoubtedly, there are important emotional, personality, and learned behavior factors that contribute to constipation. Parents reward their children for successful bowel action and imbue in many of them the idea that daily movements are essential for cleanliness and purity. Sigmund Freud attributed repression of defecation to anal eroticism. If the patient is an unmarried woman, it has been said that marriage will effect a cure, but I know of no controlled trials to substantiate this!

In colon inertia, the rectum is often full and the defecation reflex is ignored. Children, businessmen, and travelers, unable to fit a trip to the toilet into their busy schedules, habitually retain feces and stifle the defecation reflex. In his book on constipation published in 1909, Hertz, with a burst of Edwardian chauvinism, declared that

> women who have the whole morning before them with nothing of great importance to do, often put off the unpleasant duty until the inclination to defecate has disappeared. This is particularly likely to occur if they remain in bed for breakfast.

Perhaps to escape the wrath of suffragettes, the author changed his name to *Hurst* at the time of his 1919 edition! If the urge to defecate is repeatedly ignored, the bowel accommodates, and the individual eventually loses the awareness of a full rectum.

It is not surprising that many constipated patients use laxatives. In some instances of colonic inertia or megacolon, the colon damage has been attributed to chronic laxative use or abuse, but it is not always certain which came first (see Chapter 19). Drugs implicated in constipation are discussed in Chapter 20.

CLINICAL MANIFESTATIONS

The characteristic stools of the irritable bowel have been discussed previously. In colonic inertia or megacolon the hypotonic colon produces infrequent voluminous stools, which are often liquified as a result of purgatives or decomposition during their long transit. Paradoxically, diarrhea may occur in impacted patients, a situation not recognized unless digital rectal examination is performed. Only fluid finds its way around the solid fecal mass in the rectum. In addition, anal sphincter function may be impaired by a large fecal mass pressing from above with resulting incontinence.

The individual with constipation may complain of headache, foul breath, furred tongue, loss of appetite, flatulence, irritability, and insomnia. Many patients have a vague, indescribable sense of unease or ill health when constipated, and are greatly relieved by defecation. Early in this century, Arbuthnot Lane, a British orthopedic surgeon, attributed these symptoms to "chronic intestinal stasis." He believed that absorption of toxins from the colon led to such disparate conditions as depression, premature senility, changes of vision, and falling hair. In fact, since the middle ages, many illnesses have been blamed on colon stasis. This fanciful process has been called *autointoxication*. To prevent this self-poisoning, Lane led a campaign to stamp out colons. Incredible as it seems, Lane's views had considerable influence and reinforced the ritual purging that continues to this day.

Before Lane, nineteenth-century European writers felt that the colon was a useless and dangerous "encumbrance." One author declared that "every child should have its large intestine and its appendix surgically removed when 2 or 3 years of age." Such was the disrepute to which the poor colon had fallen by the twentieth century.

Lane's disciples believed, without a shred of evidence other than his testimony, that one stool a day was insufficient. Some of them advocated a vegetarian natural diet that contained whole wheat bread and bran porridge, because of its fermentative and bowel-opening effects. Thus, the high-fiber diet of today has some roots in Lane's theories, but few fiber proponents will admit to any association, which is a valuable lesson. Those who believe fiber to be beneficial to bowel function should take care not to discredit the fiber hypothesis by prematurely attributing all sorts of non-colonic diseases to fiber deficiency. The line between science and humbug is not always obvious.

To disprove the autointoxication theory, five healthy men were required to eat normally but refrain from defecation for 90 hours. Eventually, each man complained of symptoms of "acute intoxication," such as coated tongue, foul breath, mental sluggishness, and headache; they also became depressed, restless, and irritable. All subjects experienced immediate relief following an enema, which seems to militate against toxemia. Thus, the symptoms are now believed to be due to distension. In fact, masses of cotton wool packed into the rectum produce identical effects. Nonetheless, the concept of colon cleanliness has roots deep in our culture. Even with empty colons, some individuals insist that their many vague symptoms are due to constipation and ritually purge themselves.

DIAGNOSIS

First of all, the physician needs to establish that a person complaining of constipation is indeed constipated. This diagnosis requires careful evaluation of the frequency of defecation, consistency of the stool, and effort required to defecate. Two rough guidelines have been used in clinical surveys: less than 3 bowel movements per week, and straining at stool on more than 75 percent of occasions.

Next, organic disease must be excluded, and this demands a careful history and physical examination. Previous surgery or nervous system injury have obvious implications. Recent onset of constipation demands rigorous exclusion of local and systemic disease, particularly carcinoma of the colon, hypothyroidism, and depression. Pus or blood in the stool should alert the physician to the possibility of organic disease. Blood mixed with the stool almost certainly indicates important colon disease. Blood streaking the surface of the stool may be due to such local lesions as anal fissures, hemorrhoids, or proctitis, but it is dangerous to assume this. Cancer or colitis may lurk higher up.

The irritable bowel may be recognized by the features discussed in Chapter 13. As in all functional disorders, the patient's psychosocial past may be very important.

Upon examination, the alert physician should detect signs of contributing organic disease, such as anemia, hypothyroidism, or weight loss. The origin of any abdominal scars should be ascertained: Was there previous bowel surgery, or hysterectomy? Signs of obstruction should be carefully sought. A loaded colon may be palpable. A discrete irregular mass may suggest a carcinoma, particularly if it is accompanied by a large tumor-filled liver.

On digital examination of the rectum, the physician should note the presence or absence of feces. Fecal impaction, fissures, or obstructing lesions may be detected. When the subject bears down, rectal prolapse or rectocele may be observed. If the sphincter tightens during straining, anismus or a spastic pelvic floor may be suspected. Scybala suggest a spastic colon. Black stools may be due to iron or bismuth, both of which constipate. Stools may also be discolored by blood. Chalky stools suggest calcium ingestion or a recent barium examination.

Sigmoidoscopy should be performed in all cases of constipation to exclude rectal disease (see Chapter 22). Spasm of the lower sigmoid may be observed in a spastic colon, and a toneless, dilated rectosigmoid may be observed in a hypotonic one. Melanosis coli is evidence of cathartic abuse (Chapter 19). Most patients who are over 40 should have a barium enema examination and hemoglobin estimation.

Special Tests

Serial plain x-rays of the abdomen with or without ingested radio-opaque markers may help the physician judge progress of stool through the colon during treatment or in those individuals with denied defecation. Most pediatric centers have an apparatus for measuring sphincter relaxation in response to rectal distension. If failure of the sphincter to relax leads to suspicion of Hirschsprung's disease, deep rectal and anal biopsies may be done to find the denervated segment.

TREATMENT

General Measures

Little can be done about one's age or sex, but the sufferer of constipation can do much to alter many of the contributing environmental factors and personal habits that are described above. Constipating drugs should be avoided whenever possible. As repeatedly pointed out, laxatives are not a good solution to constipation: at best, they are ineffective in the treatment of colonic inertia; at worst, they force peristalsis against an obstructing anorectal angle or damage nerve plexuses (Chapter 19). In most cases, a high-fiber diet employing bran or psyllium along with extra fluids is the cornerstone of management (Chapter 13). Sometimes very large doses of bran are required: up to 9 tablespoonfuls per day. Rarely, too much bran with insufficient fluids, or dehydration may cause obstruction. Regular exercise according to the person's physical state is also very helpful. At the very least, a constipated individual should embark upon daily brisk walks.

Constipation often results from enforced confinement to bed, such as after a heart attack, especially if the patient must grapple with pulleys in order to be aligned with a bedpan. A bedside commode is much less strenuous and ensures a more physiologic position.

The patient should try to retrain the atonic, constipated colon—a goal that is best achieved by using natural reflexes to advantage. The resting colon may be spurred into action by a meal, particularly breakfast. Many individuals insist that their bowels function only following a customary morning coffee or cigarette, although whether this effect is pharmacologic, physiologic, or psychologic is uncertain. Regular postprandial retirement with a good book to the relaxing solitude of the toilet may also have a salutary effect. One early writer (Gant, 1909), however, described reading at stool as a "pernicious habit and a common source of constipation because it diverts the mind." Perhaps it depends on what is read! The constipated of the Western world are unlikely to be persuaded to adopt the squat position, but a low toilet seat results in a position more favorable for defecation. Placing a box under the feet may achieve the same effect. Comfortable surroundings are essential if toilet retraining is to be successful. Certainly, a cold drafty outhouse is no place to commence the exercise.

To initiate bowel activity in those accustomed to taking laxatives, it may be necessary to use an enema or osmotic agent, such as lactulose or milk of magnesia. A glycerine suppository, while inactive pharmacologically, helps stimulate the defecation reflex. Attention to such details, along with the use of bran, may restore even the most recalcitrant colon to normalcy. If all else fails, regular osmotic laxatives or skillfully administered isotonic saline enemas are less likely to further damage the gut wall with chronic use than is a stimulant laxative.

Psychotherapy

Psychological features must also be considered. In the irritable bowel syndrome with constipation, the patient's psychosocial situation should be explored. Reassurance that no serious disease is present is not enough; the patient must be allowed to ventilate his or her problems. The physician should then point out how such problems may exacerbate gut dysfunction.

In some women with constipation, there may be a contributing sexual dysfunction that may require the assistance of a skilled therapist or gynecologist. In such cases, depression should be sought and, if discovered, treated as the primary disease. If possible, phobias or obsessions about defecation should be dealt with. Some patients may be so timorous of defecation that they will travel great distances just to use their own toilet; others may refuse to defecate when there is anyone in the house.

Surgery

Although colectomy for constipation is certainly out of fashion, it does not follow that surgeons have lost all interest in the operation. Attempts to surgically correct the motor abnormalities described above have generally met with dismal failure. In at least one half of those undergoing colon removal for colonic inertia, further surgery is necessary because of small-bowel obstruction. Most surgeons have abandoned this line of work, and no patient should submit to such surgery without expert advice.

Other Measures

There is some enthisiasm for biofeedback in selected cases. In the spastic pelvic floor syndrome, for example, the patient may, by means of a device screening his or her own anal pressure on a television monitor, attempt to relax, rather than contract, the pelvic muscles during defecation. Although this procedure seems harmless enough, like hypnotherapy and behavior modification it requires more study.

SUMMARY

Any definition of constipation must take into account the frequency, consistency, and the ease of passage of stools, as well as the patient's attitude toward them. Organic disease must be excluded, particularly in the presence of bleeding or recent onset. Most constipation is associated with the irritable bowel syndrome and responds well to fiber and to reassurance. Colonic inertia, spastic pelvic floor, megacolon, and denied defecation pose special problems. Important considerations in a patient include age, sex, childbirth, hysterectomy, dehydration, fiber lack, drug and laxative use, inactivity and disability, faulty habits or position at defecation, and emotion. Sound diagnosis depends upon history and colon examination. Special tests increase our understanding of intractable cases somewhat, but seldom lead to definitive therapy. Successful treatment consists of measures to correct the contributing factors. In general, drugs and surgery have little place in the management of constipation.

CHAPTER SEVENTEEN

Proctalgia Fugax
A Real Pain in the Ass

In a hospital corridor, a 49-year-old woman suddenly fell to the floor in agony. Two nurses found her doubled up and speechless with rectal pain. Fearing that she was suffering a seizure, they called for help. Fortunately, she recovered sufficiently to wave off cardiac resuscitation. She was shortly assisted to her feet and went home, none the worse for her brief ordeal.

The first attack of rectal pain had occurred 14 years previously. Since then she had experienced one or two bouts per year. The excruciating pain, centered above the anal canal, occurred mainly at night, with no obvious precipitating activity. It began abruptly and ceased equally abruptly, having lasted several minutes. Between attacks she suffered no bowel symptoms. There was no abnormality of the anus or rectum.

This patient was greatly relieved to learn that she had suffered from *proctalgia fugax*. How reassuring to have such a euphonious and authoritative sobriquet applied to an affliction that one has suffered anonymously with for years. The term is actually a curious hybrid of Latin and Greek and was coined by T. E. H. Thaysen, a Scandinavian who most likely spoke neither language. Proctalgia fugax may be defined as a sudden, severe pain in the rectal region, lasting several seconds or minutes, which then disappears completely with no sequela and no pathologic abnormality.

The first recognized case was reported by A. S. Myrtle in 1883 in the *British Medical Journal*. He described rectal pain as "very fitful in its attacks, coming on at long intervals." The victim "will go to bed perfectly well and awake at any hour with a gnawing pain in the sphincter." His patient's worst attack occurred as he was entering a railway carriage and was relieved when he sat on a foot-warmer provided by British Rail for first-class passengers. Myrtle, however, offers no advice for those traveling second class.

EPIDEMIOLOGY

Few doctors are aware of proctalgia fugax unless they have it themselves, and even then they may not be able to name it. Yet sufferers are a numerous, if taciturn, lot. In our 1980 survey of 301 apparently healthy British people, 41 (14 percent) admitted to having this symptom, which compares to 18 percent of 167 young American hospital workers who had cramplike or spasmodic anorectal pain. None of these individuals had sought medical attention. H. Ibrahim found proctalgia in 4 percent of those presenting to a student surgical clinic with rectal complaints, and in only 0.5 percent of 1,024 private cases with rectal complaints. However, most sufferers do not volunteer that they suffer from this rude and evanescent symptom. Among 148 patients with gastrointestinal complaints who were asked, one third admitted to it. It is said that proctalgia has a tendency to occur in families, but with an overall prevalence rate of 14 percent, and an even higher prevalence among patients, any family association may be coincidental.

Since many astonished physicians describe their own attacks anonymously in medical journals, the belief arose that this phenomenon occurred largely in tense young men. One author has even termed it "the doctor's disease." However, in our population study, proctalgia fugax occurred in 18 percent of 164 women and only 9 percent of 137 men. Among 148 gastroenterology patients seen in my clinic, the prevalence was 51 percent in females and 12 percent in males. The prevalence of proctalgia seems to decrease with age. Some elderly subjects remember suffering attacks of rectal pain in their youth. This phenomenon is not confined to adults. Sir Arthur Hurst, the distinguished physiologist, described it in a 15-year-old boy, and I attended a 7-year-old with the typical syndrome.

In addition to the surveys that were performed in Britain, the United States, and Canada, there are also descriptions from continental Europe. Reports from Russia and Egypt indicate the occurrence of proctalgia on both sides of the Iron Curtain and in the Third World.

CLINICAL DESCRIPTION

Most sufferers report that proctalgia pain is severe. Those in a position to compare, rank the pain with biliary colic or childbirth. Fainting may even occur. However, because the pain is so common, and so few report it to the doctor, it seems likely that severity varies greatly. In the Canadian patient series, only one half of those reporting proctalgia were forced to interrupt their activities during an attack, and 8 percent were "in agony." Usually, the pain is located in the midline, somewhere above the anal sphincter. Although the pain may be unilateral, it seldom travels elsewhere.

In most sufferers, proctalgia attacks occur less than 6 times in a year. In the 49 patients with gastrointestinal disease who also had proctalgia, most recalled that attacks lasted less than a minute, and 90 percent said they lasted less than 5 minutes. Only 2 patients endured it more than 30 minutes.

About 1 patient in 10 suffers exclusively at night, and one quarter both day and night. Attacks may occur after defecation in 30 to 40 percent of individuals. Despite reports that attacks follow various types of sexual activity, it is a relief to hear that 94 percent escape such retribution. Several individuals report that attacks are likely to occur during fatigue or stress, and one correspondent could willfully provoke an attack by undertaking boring, undesirable work. Another individual, a lawyer, endured proctalgia attacks in court, which certainly must have impressed the jury. Some individuals suffer attacks out of the blue. Hurst described a British soldier who fainted on parade during an attack; stiff upper lip indeed! One man, stricken at a party, was seen to retire to a bedroom, remove his shoe, fold his leg under him on a chair, and sit with his heel pressed tightly against his anus. He had 10 relatives with the same affliction, but we are uncertain if they all assumed the same posture for relief. Some individuals report that proctalgia attacks occur with heat, others with cold. One man even claimed that he could predict the weather, since his pain was triggered by a cold east wind.

Cause, precipitating events, and cure may be argued, but there is little disagreement among sufferers about the nature of proctalgia pain itself. It commences suddenly in the anal area, building rapidly to a peak, then eases off, leaving the victim weary but well. To some, it may seem to last a very long time, but scant seconds or minutes are recorded on the clock. Cramping, stabbing, aching, grinding, and gnawing are the words used to describe the sensation. One sufferer offers this vivid description; "dull, throbbing, tearing, sickening pain comparable to nothing on earth—one feels as though a hard stone in the rectum was wanting to get out." Another sufferer likened it to a wedge "shot into the anus."

Some victims describe a slight warning or "aura" in which there may be a sensation of weariness, or a dull abdominal discomfort prior to an attack. Others notice that relief of pain coincides with the passage of flatus. Between paroxysms, there are no anorectal symptoms.

There is no doubt that proctalgia fugax can be debilitating. One sufferer has written:

> Recently, I was diagnosed as having "proctalgia fugax." This diagnosis came after suffering 6 years, seeing 13 different doctors, undergoing 2 operations (hysterectomy, hemorrhoidectomy) and spending thousands of dollars on laboratory tests, consults and x-rays. Not one . . . was able to diagnose this malady. I had to travel 250 miles . . . for a diagnosis. . . . I was very happy to hear that there was a name for my buttocks' pain, but disappointed that at this time nothing could be done. . . . These attacks can occur right after urinating, during orgasm or out of a clear blue sky. You live in fear because you never know when one can strike you. They can last from 10 minutes to 2 hours. The severity ranges from moderate pain to excruciating. . . . This prob-

lem has disabled me both physically and mentally. . . . I gave up a
rewarding position.

Fortunately, such an extreme case is rare.

MECHANISMS

The cause of proctalgia fugax is unknown, so theories flourish.
In his monograph on constipation published in 1909, Hurst suggested that spasm of the sphincter may occur in association with
spasm elsewhere in the colon. However, physicians who have examined themselves during an attack report a lax anal sphincter.
Others have noted a tender band on one or the other side of the
rectum which they took to be the muscles of the pelvic floor (see
Figure 8). The relief with perineal pressure, the location of pain
often to one side of the rectum, the lack of relationship to bowel
action, and the failure of smooth-muscle-relaxing drugs to relieve
it all point to a disorder of striated muscle. Thus, the pain might
be thought of as a cramp, such as one might experience in the
muscle of a limb.

One physician had occasion to examine a patient with a sigmoidoscope during a proctalgia attack. He noticed an enlarged
prostate, engorged rectal veins, a red mucosa, and a palpable,
tender pelvic floor. In a French study, researchers also noted dilated rectal veins in 5 patients they examined with arteriography.
However, this report does not square with another physician's
apparently normal sigmoidoscopic examination of two patients
during an attack. He, in turn, observed that episodes of pain appeared to coincide with rectosigmoid colon contractions. It seems
likely that these are epiphenomena. Glimpses of the anorectum
during an attack of proctalgia fugax must require infinite patience
and good luck.

At the Mayo Clinic, 48 patients with proctalgia fugax were
submitted to psychological and personality testing. Many of these
patients were found to be perfectionists, and were anxious, tense,
hypochondriacal, and had had neurotic symptoms in childhood.

Furthermore, the authors stated that intelligent, anxious, and perfectionist persons focus on pain and somatize emotional conflicts. At this point, many readers will suspect that the above characteristics are those of people who go to doctors with seemingly minor complaints. But it is well to remember that most of those who suffer this commonplace disorder do not seek medical help. The Mayo Clinic study did not employ controls, and since the patients were no doubt highly selected by the time they were referred there, no conclusions therefore can be drawn.

RELATIONSHIP OF PROCTALGIA FUGAX TO THE IRRITABLE BOWEL SYNDROME

The same Mayo Clinic group described above also reported that functional gastrointestinal disorders occurred in 52 percent of their proctalgia fugax patients. We have already seen, however, that these patients may be a special, complaining subgroup. In another survey of 301 nonpatient subjects, symptoms associated with the irritable bowel syndrome (IBS) were indeed more common in those reporting proctalgia than in those without it. However, this association may not be unique to the IBS. Among my 198 patients, proctalgia had a similar occurrence in those with peptic ulcer, inflammatory bowel disease, and IBS. It could be that those with gut complaints have a heightened awareness and greater recall for proctalgia.

It also seems possible that these two common functional disorders have a common etiology. It should be remembered, however, that the IBS appears to be due to altered smooth muscle function or sensitivity in the large *and* small bowel, whereas proctalgia fugax is believed to be due to spasm of pelvic floor *striated* muscle. Although I have chosen to consider proctalgia, like the IBS, as part of the irritable gut spectrum, it seems unlikely that these two conditions are fundamentally related.

DIAGNOSIS

A diagnosis of proctalgia fugax can be made from the history of infrequent attacks of very severe, deep, nonradiating rectal pain, occurring after bowel movements, after coitus, or spontaneously. The pain may onset day or night, ceasing abruptly in less than 10 to 20 minutes. Unless the physician happens to come upon a victim during such a paroxysm, no clinical signs can be expected. Sweating, fainting, and tight, tender pelvic floor muscles may be observed during such an attack. Congested rectal veins or altered gut motility are not reliable or specific features.

On the other hand, an anal fissure may be the cause of sharp anal pain during defecation. In such cases, the stool may be hard and streaked with blood. Usually, a tiny tear is found when the physician carefully inspects the anus. A thrombosed hemorrhoid should also be painfully obvious. In the past, anal pain has been attributed to advanced syphilis, but in this case the pain lasts for hours, and may radiate and be associated with a painful urge to defecate. Pain localized to the tip of the spine and aggravated by sitting is called *coccydynia*. There is often a history of injury. High rectal pain with fever may result from an inflamed prostate in males or pelvic infection in females.

Rectal neuralgia lasts longer than proctalgia, radiates to the sacrum, and is of a burning nature. Persistent anal pain without any explanation can occur and might be called *status proctalgia*. Most likely, it is psychogenic in nature.

TREATMENT

The great variety and inventiveness of treatments confessed by physician sufferers attest to the lack of general satisfaction with any one form of treatment. Some prefer heat, others cold. Many sufferers get relief by distending the rectum with air, fluid, or even glycerine and carry enema equipment for this purpose. Still others dilate the anal canal with their finger, whereas others prefer pressure on the anus. Assumption of the knee to chest position, or a doubled-up squat, has also been advocated. During an attack, some individuals prefer to sit on the edge of a hard seat, on something hot, on a foot, or on a toilet reading something interesting. Others believe that they can break an attack by eating or drinking to stimulate the gastrocolonic response. One correspondent reported that a constantly suffering colleague noted immediate cessation of attacks when he discontinued cigarettes. Like Mark Twain, he found it so easy to stop smoking that he did it many times and abolished his proctalgia each time. For those whose attacks follow sex, the treatment should be equally straightforward.

Attacks of proctalgia, which seem to be an eternity to the sufferer, are actually fleeting. Nine out of 10 patients report that the pain lasts less than 5 minutes. Therefore, no drug, unless administered intravenously or inhaled at the beginning of an attack, could be expected to influence the pain. However, the rapid, spontaneous cessation of pain may leave the patient with the erroneous impression that any drug he has used is effective; otherwise, how else can one explain the advocacy of neurotrasentin phenobarbitol, or propantheline. Inhalants, such as chloroform or amyl nitrite, are either unacceptable or unsuccessful. Since quinine may help prevent leg cramps, it has been suggested as a proctalgia prophylaxis. A Russian author, M. B. Barkar, recommends a presacral Novocain block with the administration of penicillin, streptomycin, and hydrocortisone paralleled by a treatment with microenemas containing 0.5 percent novocaine and cod liver oil. Should a confession of cure not follow, we can presume that there is a gulag for stubborn cases.

Some people appear to have attacks that are sufficiently severe to warrant treatment, if such were available. For the reasons given, no drug can be recommended for acute attacks other than a mild pain tablet. Nervous people should be reassured that no serious condition, especially cancer, exists, and that the attacks seem to become less frequent with age. It is logical to treat any accompanying irritable bowel, if present, with a high-bulk diet since an effortless bowel movement might be less likely to trigger an attack. One should withdraw drugs that might have an adverse gut effect. However, as Thaysen has concluded, proctalgia fugax must be considered "harmless, unpleasant, and incurable."

SUMMARY

Proctalgia fugax is a recurrent, sudden, severe, deep-seated supra-anal pain usually lasting less than 5 minutes, occurring night or day, afflicting females more than males, sometimes precipitated by defecation or sexual activity, and ceasing abruptly without trace. Attacks occur several times a year in 10 to 20 percent of the population, and seem to decrease with age. The pain is believed to be due to spasm of the pelvic floor muscles. Usually, there is little difficulty in distinguishing the pain of proctalgia from that of coccydynia or anal fissure.

The profusion of remedies that are recommended for the relief of proctalgia bespeaks the inefficacy of any of them. The anxious, often cancerphobic patient needs reassurance that is best provided by a complete history, physical examination, and sigmoidoscopy. Further treatment is generally of little avail, because the attack is usually over before any drug can act. Many sufferers find relief by exerting warm pressure against the anus, which, at least, is something that can easily be done.

PART THREE

Topics Important to Those with Gut Reactions

CHAPTER EIGHTEEN

Diverticula

Diverticular disease of the colon is very common in Western societies. Indeed, one half of the population of Europe, North America, and Australia can expect to acquire diverticula as they reach 60 or 70 years of age. Although diverticular disease is rare among the Bantu, Africans who adopt a Western life-style can become liable. Its prevalence is reduced among certain Westerners, such as vegetarians and wartime Britons, who eat a fiber-rich diet. As a result of these observations, this "disease of Western civilization" is widely believed to be due to a fiber-deficient diet.

Fortunately, most people with diverticular disease (diverticulosis coli) suffer no serious consequences. A minority, however, have complications that in the United States result annually in 200,000 hospitalizations and more than $.75 billion in health care costs. Diverticular disease may be complicated by hemorrhage or diverticulitis (perforation of a diverticulum with infection). In this chapter we will discuss the clinical features and management of uncomplicated diverticular disease. Complicated diverticular disease will be briefly described to emphasize its difference from the simple presence of diverticula.

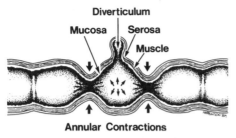

Diverticulum

Mucosa | **Serosa**

Muscle

Annular Contractions

Figure 25. Formation of colon diverticula. Neighboring contractions of the colon generate increased intraluminal pressure within a segment that forces the mucosa through a defect in the gut wall adjacent to the nutrient artery where it pierces the gut wall. It is believed the Western low-fiber diet results in a narrower lumen, permitting higher pressures to be generated (Laplace's law) (see Chapter 6). See also Figure 26.

WHAT ARE DIVERTICULA?

Where a nutrient blood vessel pierces the colon wall, there is a tiny defect or interruption in the integrity of the muscular layer. Presumably, as a result of increased intraluminal pressure, the mucosal layer may be forced through the defect to form a bulge or sac (Figures 25 and 26). (For those whose Latin is rusty, one sac is a *diverticulum* and more than one are *diverticula*.) From the point of view of the complications of diverticular disease, it is important to recognize that (1) the nutrient blood vessel is stretched over the bulge and may bleed into the lumen, and (2) the sac has no muscle layer and is liable to perforate with resulting infection (Table 26).

Table 26
Diverticular Disease

A. Uncomplicated diverticular disease
B. Complicated diverticular disease
  1. Diverticular hemorrhage
  2. Diverticulitis:
    a. Peridiverticulitis
    b. Intra-abdominal abscess
    c. Fistulas
    d. Bowel obstruction
    e. Peritonitis

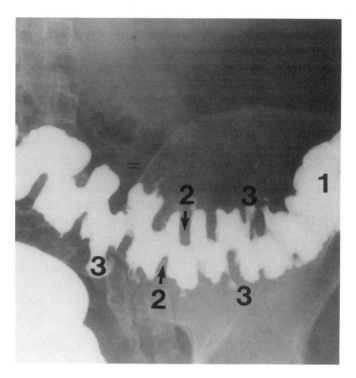

Figure 26. A barium examination of the large bowel showing diverticula in the descending and sigmoid colon: (1) barium in sigmoid colon; (2) annular contractions; and (3) diverticula.

UNCOMPLICATED DIVERTICULAR DISEASE (DIVERTICULOSIS)

Relationship to the Irritable Bowel

Many, perhaps most, individuals with colon diverticula suffer no gastrointestinal symptoms. In 1925, two physicians, Spriggs and Marxor, noted that 71 of 100 patients with x-ray-proven diverticulosis had flatulence, abdominal pain or discomfort often related to defecation, diarrhea, constipation, or alternating diarrhea and constipation, which are all easily recognized as features of the irritable bowel syndrome (IBS). It has therefore been suggested that the irritable bowel is a prediverticular state. Almy has asked, "Are diverticulosis and the irritable colon independent or related processes?"

Against a direct relationship is the observation that of 521 patients found to have diverticular disease on x-ray, more than one half had symptoms less than once a month. Furthermore, many patients with diverticular disease are asymptomatic and have colon motility tracings indistinguishable from normals. However, those complaining of abdominal pain, distension, and irregular bowel habit seem to have sigmoid motility features similar to those with the IBS. Balloon distension of the rectum produces similar pressure responses in subjects with symptomatic diverticular disease and the IBS.

We have seen that colon diverticula appear to be present in more than one half of elderly Westerners. Abdominal pain and/or altered bowel habit is present in about one third of apparently healthy adults in Britain and in the United States. This prevalence is similar in young, middle-aged, and elderly patients, although constipation is more common in the old. It is not surprising then that the two phenomena, IBS and diverticula, may coexist in many older people (Figure 27). Fiber deficiency and colon motility disturbances may be important in both groups, but it is apparent that diverticulosis coli and the IBS may manifest themselves quite independently.

Among patients presenting to a gastroenterology clinic in Bristol, England, complaining of abdominal pain with or without altered bowel habit, those with the IBS were compared with those who had organic gastrointestinal disease (see Chapter 13). The IBS patients were found more likely to have abdominal pain relieved with defecation, altered consistency and frequency of bowel movements with the onset of pain, abdominal distension, mucus in the stool, and a feeling of incomplete evacuation (Table 13). These symptoms have been described in other IBS populations and are very common in apparently healthy people.

In Ottawa, we administered a questionnaire to 97 outpatients

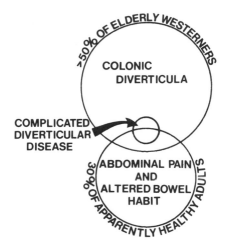

Figure 27. Relationships of IBS, uncomplicated diverticular disease, and complicated diverticular disease.

who were referred for air contrast barium enema. The x-ray was interpreted by a radiologist, who did not know the results of the questionnaire. Forty-nine had normal x-rays and 27 had uncomplicated diverticular disease. The six symptoms described above were similarly prevalent in both groups (Table 27). Even weight loss, rectal bleeding, and abdominal pain at night were found equally in individuals with and without diverticula. In a study from a radiology practice in New Zealand, abdominal pain, diarrhea, and constipation were equally present in 100 patients with diverticular disease and 138 patients with normal x-rays. These two studies thus demonstrate that no symptoms can be considered characteristic of uncomplicated diverticular disease. In both reports, all patients with diverticula had sigmoid involvement. Therefore, it is possible that IBS symptoms occur only among patients with sigmoid diverticular disease, perhaps in association with muscular hypertrophy. More likely, the IBS occurs commonly and coincidentally with all types of diverticula, even those in the cecum.

Table 27
Incidence of Bowel Symptoms in Subjects with Uncomplicated
Diverticular Disease Compared to Those with Normal Barium Enema[a]

Symptoms	Diverticular disease (n = 27)	Normal barium enema (n = 49)	Significance of difference
Weight loss >5 lbs in 3 months	4 (14.8)	9 (18.4)	NS[c]
Rectal bleeding	10 (37)	20 (41)	NS
Abdominal pain > 6× in year	17 (63)	30 (61.2)	NS
Night pain	8 (47.1)	11 (36.7)	NS
Pain relieved with defecation[b]			
Ever	11 (64.7)	14 (46.7)	NS
Often	11 (64.7)	12 (40)	NS
Altered stool frequency with	4 (23.5)	7 (23.3)	NS
onset of pain or more frequent stools with onset of pain[b]	4 (23.5)	4 (13.3)	NS
Altered stool consistency with	6 (35.2)	11 (36.7)	NS
onset of pain or looser stools in onset of pain[b]	6 (35.2)	7 (23.3)	NS
Abdominal distension[b]			
Ever	19 (70.4)	26 (53.1)	NS
Often	12 (44.7)	13 (26.1)	NS
Feeling of incomplete evacuation after defecation[b]			
Ever	18 (66.6)	32 (66.6)	NS
Often	6 (22.2)	18 (36.7)	NS
Mucus in stool[b]			
Ever	9 (33.3)	17 (34.7)	NS
Often	4 (14.8)	5 (10.2)	NS
Straining at stool more than 25% of time	5 (18.5)	8 (16.3)	NS
Loose watery stools more than 25% of time	4 (14.8)	6 (12.2)	NS
Proctalgia fugax	6 (22.2)	9 (18.7)	NS
Laxative use	8 (29.6)	17 (34.9)	NS

[a] Reproduced with permission of *Digestive Diseases and Sciences* (1982;27:605–608). Figures in parentheses indicate percentage of total (n).
[b] Symptoms characteristic of the irritable bowel syndrome (Chapter 13).
[c] NS = not significantly different.

These data support the notion that when bowel symptoms occur with diverticulosis coli, they may be due to a coexistent irritable bowel rather than to the diverticular process itself. Yet it is possible that they have a common etiology. In this context, it should be noted that IBS symptoms are prevalent in patients with peptic ulcer and inflammatory bowel disease, and that this does not imply a causal relationship.

MANAGEMENT OF UNCOMPLICATED DIVERTICULAR DISEASE

Asymptomatic patients need no treatment, but those with IBS symptoms should be managed as outlined in Chapter 13. First, the patient with colon diverticula needs reassurance that no grave illness exists. It may be that fear of cancer or other serious disease led to the barium enema which revealed the diverticula in the first place.

There have been 4 placebo-controlled trials of the use of bran in the treatment of uncomplicated diverticular disease (Table 16). The symptoms being treated were presumably those of the IBS, and, in some studies, symptomatic patients with and without diverticula are lumped together. It appears that 20 to 30 grams of bran is necessary if a therapeutic effect is to be achieved. In a 1977 study by Brogribb, less pain and a lower total symptom score was achieved with the use of bran biscuits. However, this improvement was most marked at 3 months, suggesting that continued use of bran is important. Although Ornstein, in his study in 1981, did not achieve an overall beneficial effect at 16 weeks, the initial pain score in his patients was very low, and only 7 grams of daily dietary fiber was used. There have been 3 placebo-controlled trials of pharmaceutical bulking agents in the treatment of diverticular disease, with methyl cellulose appearing to be ineffective. Isbaghula and psyllium produced results similar to those of the bran studies. Sufficient dose and length of treatment seem to be important.

Although the trials of bran and other bulking agents fail to show any clear benefit, bran is used for the IBS by most gastroenterologists in Britain and in the United States (see Chapter 13). Therefore, it seems logical to advise its use in symptomatic uncomplicated diverticular disease as well. As in the case of the irritable bowel, those patients with uncomplicated diverticular disease and IBS symptoms can expect to have them for long periods of their lives. Therefore, the use of antispasmodics or other unproven pharmacotherapeutic agents seems inadvisable.

COMPLICATED DIVERTICULAR DISEASE

The complications of diverticular disease are not functional disorders. But there is a need to clarify the difference between the harmless presence of diverticula (diverticulosis) and the morbid results of rupture of a blood vessel in a diverticulum (diverticular hemorrhage) or perforation of the diverticulum itself (diverticulitis). The consequences of these events are summarized in Table 26. Again it is important to stress that complications occur in only a small number of those individuals with diverticula.

On the other hand, diverticular hemorrhage may be life-threatening and diverticulitis may result in several clinical problems. Peridiverticulitis is a situation in which the contents of the burst diverticulum are localized by body defenses to the tissues adjacent to the colon. It may present in a manner similar to that of an acute appendix with the pain on the left rather than on the right side of the abdomen. It is usually successfully treated by intravenous fluids and antibiotics. The development of an intra-abdominal abscess, drainage into another organ such as the bladder (fistula), and obstruction of the colon usually require surgery. Peritonitis, resulting from release of infected material into the abdominal cavity, is a surgical emergency.

PREVENTION

If Africans, wartime Britons, and vegetarians on high-fiber diets do not get diverticular disease, may we not prevent the disorder by prescribing fiber? There are so many different types of fiber and so many other factors that differentiate the average Westerner from the Bantu that a high-bulk diet for everybody cannot be recommended without more studies. We have seen that the type of fiber eaten by natives is quite different from that likely to be consumed by Westerners (Chapter 7). Furthermore, there is no bran in the typical African diet.

Nevertheless, we have also seen that a high-fiber diet is beneficial in symptomatic, uncomplicated diverticular disease. Further, a British study suggests that among those who already have diverticula, complications and recurrences of diverticulitis are reduced with a high-fiber diet. It does seem reasonable, therefore, to recommend a high-fiber diet to those who have symptomatic, uncomplicated diverticular disease (ie, with IBS), or to those who have suffered a complication in the past. However, it is not possible to justify either a search for diverticula in the asymptomatic population or a crusade to put fiber back in Western menus.

SUMMARY

Uncomplicated diverticular disease is usually asymptomatic. When abdominal pain or discomfort related to defecation, altered bowel habit, and flatulence occur, they are more than likely to be the result of a coexistent irritable bowel. Nonetheless, in a small number of patients, diverticula are subject to the serious complications of hemorrhage and intra-abdominal infection. Although there is insufficient evidence to justify a high-fiber diet for the general population, those individuals with diverticula and the IBS or previous complications may obtain some benefit.

CHAPTER NINETEEN

Catharsis

Find her disease
And purge it to pristine health.

Shakespeare, *Macbeth* (5.3)

It is a sobering fact that many people purge themselves because they think they are constipated. In one study, 14 of 24 patients habitually using laxatives for constipation were able to maintain a satisfactory bowel habit during a 2-week period on placebo. Other patients may purge themselves in secret, deriving who knows what pleasure from baffling their doctors with the ensuing diarrhea. For these reasons, the physician must determine whether or not the patient is indeed constipated. Bowel retraining and dietary fiber are the treatments of choice. Laxatives are seldom indicated on a chronic basis and should be reserved for the preparation of the bowel for special procedures, or episodes of constipation that occur with illness or enforced bedrest.

Constipation may be disquieting. Empires have trembled at the prospect of a laxative shortage. In a nineteenth-century exercise of pharmacologic warfare, Britain placed an embargo on the export of purgatives to Napoléon-controlled Europe. Sydney Smith satirized this costive instrument of foreign policy thus:

> What a sublime thought that no purge can now be taken between the Weser and the Garonne; that the bustling pestle is still, the canorous mortar mute, and the bowels of men locked up for fourteen degrees of latitude. . . . Were all the powers of crudity and flatulence fully explained to his Majesty's ministers? . . . Was this great plan of conquest and constipation fully developed? . . . Without castor oil they might for some months, to be sure, have carried on a lingering war; but what can they do without bark [cascara]? . . . Depend upon it, the absence of materia medica will bring them to their senses, and the cry of Bourbon and Bolus burst forth from the Baltic to the Mediterranean. (*Lancet* 1973, Vol. 2, p. 1079)

In spite of injunctions by clinical pharmacologists against their long-term use, Americans spent $368 million for more than 120 over-the-counter laxatives in 1982. In 1973, the National Health Service in Great Britain spent £7 million to cleanse the British bowels. This is folly. Laxatives have limited use in the management of constipation, and their medical interest lies mainly in the harm they do.

Catharsis means purification, and is reminiscent of medieval superstition or of the imagined evils of "autointoxication," which enthralled medical science in the early 1900s. Three grades of purgatives are described: *laxatives, cathartics,* and *drastics. Laxatives* produce a formed movement, *cathartics* a semiformed one, and *drastics* a watery diarrhea.

Even in spite of modern medical scepticism, laxatives are still part of our heritage, and the curative effects of purging have been extolled by many great physicians. David Livingstone, the physician-explorer, while traveling on the Zambezi, attributed the relatively low mortality of his party from jungle fever to a mixture of "resin, jalap and calomel, of each 8 grains; quinine and rhubarb of each 4 grains." This concoction was followed by a dessertspoonful of salts and quinine "until the ears ring." The *Livingstone pill,* as it became known, was subsequently a fashionable nostrum along the Thames.

Table 28
Oral Laxatives

Bulking agents
  Dietary fiber
  Artificial bulking agents
    Psyllium (Metamucil)
    Methyl cellulose
Lubricants
  Mineral oil
Chemical stimulants
  Diphenolic laxatives
    Phenolphthalein (Ex-lax)
    Bisacodyl (Dulcolax)
  Anthracene glycosides
    Senna (Senokot) and cascara
  Dioctyl sodium sulphosuccinate (Colace)
  Castor oil
Osmotic laxatives
  Salines
    Sodium sulfate
    Magnesium sulfate (epsom salts)
    Magnesium hydroxide (milk of magnesia)
  Lactulose (Chronulac)
Obsolete laxatives
  Mercurous chloride
  Croton oil
  Podophyllin
  Jalap

ORAL LAXATIVES

They take in at the oriface above a medicine, equally annoying and disgustful to the bowels, which relaxing the belly drives down all before it; and this they call a purge.

Jonathan Swift, *Gulliver's Travels*

The classes of laxatives are summarized in Table 28. The traditional classification into stool softeners, stimulants, and osmotic laxatives will undoubtedly be replaced when their mechanisms of action become clearer.

BULKING AGENTS

Dietary Fiber

Dietary fiber has been discussed in Chapter 7. Bran is a practical form of natural fiber and, as frequently mentioned, is the treatment of choice for most of those individuals with constipation, the irritable bowel, and even those who have functional diarrhea.

Artificial Bulking Agents

Psyllium (Metamucil, Hydrocil, Fybogel)

Psyllium hydrophilic mucilloid is a powder derived from the seed coat of a flowering plant that is native to India. In the United Kingdom, it is known as isbaghula and has been employed as a laxative in the Orient for a millennium. The modern preparation, which omits the irritant outer coat, consists of powdered natural mucilage. Diabetics should be aware that dextrose and sucrose are used in this product as dispersing agents and that one teaspoonful delivers 12 calories. Hypertensives should not be seduced by the flavored, instant mix, which contains 240 milligrams of sodium per dose. Those with celiac disease, on the other hand, need not suffer lack of fiber since this preparation is gluten-free.

Because bran in therapeutic quantities is inconvenient, many patients prefer psyllium preparations. They are extensively employed to treat the irritable bowel, constipation, perianal disease, and diverticulosis coli. To demonstrate the advertised effect of psyllium, add one teaspoonful (5 grams) of the mucilloid to a medicine glass with sufficient water to make a total of 30 milliliters, stir, and allow the mixture to stand for a few minutes. The swelling may be 15 times the initial volume. It is said that in the gut this gelling action may soften hard, marblelike stools, or firm up diarrhea stools. The resulting movement is odorless, bulky, and glistening, a welcome respite for the constipated. This explanation may appear overly simple, since it is more than likely that the metabolic products of psyllium are involved in its laxative action. The recommended dose is 1 to 2 teaspoonfuls (5 to 10 grams) 3 times a day with meals. As with bran, psyllium may take days and sometimes weeks to take effect, and bloating may occur with the commencement of therapy. The dose should be adjusted to achieve a stool that is neither loose nor stony hard. Ten grams produces little benefit in terms of stool weight, transit time, and symptoms. The optimum dose of psyllium is 20 grams (4 teaspoonfuls per day). Thirty grams is no better than 20.

In a 1947 uncontrolled study, psyllium was found to be an effective treatment of both atonic and spastic constipation, but more so in the latter disorder. A recent, well-conducted trial demonstrated a substantial improvement in well-being in patients with the IBS who were receiving psyllium. As in other studies with bulking agents, transit time was reduced, and constipation improved. In a group of elderly, debilitated patients, psyllium gained ready acceptance when substituted for their usual laxative.

Like bran, psyllium has few disadvantages. Fecal impaction is a potential hazard in patients with an underlying obstruction. Hydration also seems to be important. Ingestion of whole psyllium seeds has caused esophageal obstruction in at least one elderly person. Some individuals who were employed in the manufacture of psyllium powder have suffered asthmatic attacks.

Other Bulking Agents

Methylcellulose is a bulking agent with little water-holding capacity and a modest effect on stool weight. It does shorten transit time, and has been recommended for its so-called demulcent effect (soothing and allaying irritation). Perhaps "roughage" should be called "smoothage." Eighty-five percent of orally administered cellulose is recovered from the small bowel, but it appears to be substantially fermented in the colon. It would appear that any laxative effect of cellulose is partly dependent on the products of this fermentation: short chain fatty acids, hydrogen, carbon dioxide, and methane. The degree of fermentation seems to vary with the purity, particle size, and source of the cellulose, and the age, transit time, and microflora of the subject. Cellulose is an active principle in bran (Chapter 6), but alone it is less effective than psyllium in the treatment of constipation.

Many other bulking agents have been offered to the constipated. The products of certain vegetable gums, such as gum arabic and karaya, are available. They attract water and form a gel that is resistant to mechanical action. Digestion by colon bacteria is unpredictable, but metabolites of these gums are thought to have a laxative effect. Their impact on nutrition is unknown, and there are certain hazards. One patient swallowed a handful of powdered gum, which lodged in the esophagus. Attempts to wash it down with water resulted in swelling and further obstruction, necessitating surgical removal. Agar, a mucilaginous product of kelp that swells in water, is combined with mineral oil in some proprietary preparations.

All things considered, if a bulking agent is required for constipation, diarrhea, or perianal disease, a high-fiber diet is best. A bran supplement is a convenient, if poorly palatable, second choice. If an individual must use an artificial bulking agent, psyllium is a smooth way to rough it.

LUBRICANTS

Mineral Oil (Liquid Paraffin)

Mineral oil was popularized in Britain by Arbuthnot Lane, who introduced it from continental Europe. This intrepid but wrongheaded enthusiast had Britons consuming 30,000 gallons of the oil annually long before the North Sea was tapped. Although this substance has some lubricating activity, it does little, if anything, to improve the physiology of defecation.

There are many reasons why this oil should not be used. In the elderly and infants, with whom it may be employed chronically, aspirated oil fails to stimulate the cough reflex. Sliding stealthily into the lung, it may cause a chemical pneumonia. The oil is a solvent for the fat-soluble vitamins A, D, E, and K, whose absorption from the gut may be impaired. It also may interfere with the healing of bowel fistulas. Oil leaking from the anus may cause pruritis ani (itchy anus), and large amounts may actually cause incontinence. For these reasons, mineral oil should be banished from the marketplace.

CHEMICAL STIMULANTS

Diphenolic Laxatives

Phenolphthalein

In the late nineteenth century, Hungarian wine was pale in comparison to its French competitor. It was discovered that phenolphthalein imparted a richer red color to the Hungarian wine and no doubt produced a popular catharsis as well. Around the turn of the century, Zoltan von Vamossy was commissioned by an alarmed government to investigate the safety of this measure. Von Vamossy administered the poorly soluble substance to subjects in his laboratory, and a highly successful commercial laxative was born. The winemaker's loss became the patent medicine industry's gain.

Phenolphthalein is poorly soluble in water, and its mode and site of cathartic action is uncertain. It is absorbed from the gut and excreted in the bile conjugated to glucuronide. The soluble glucuronide may be deconjugated to the insoluble phenolphthalein by bacteria in the colon, which is the primary site of action. Although the drug has a direct effect on the left colon muscle, this alone could not account for the production of watery stool. There appears, as well, to be inhibition of water and mineral absorption in the small bowel.

The usual dose of 100 to 200 milligrams of phenolphthalein produces one or two loose, watery stools 6 to 8 hours after ingestion. Phenolphthalein appears in several popular over-the-counter preparations, such as Ex-Lax. A 3-year-old boy survived an accidental overdose of phenolphthalein, so it must be nontoxic. Hypersensitivity reactions have been reported, including a rare encephalitis. Long-term use and abuse of the drug, however, may have devastating effects (see below). Some phenolphthalein glucuronide is excreted in the urine. When urine containing the drug is made alkaline and boiled, it becomes red, thus providing a simple means to detect surreptitious use.

Bisacodyl

Bisacodyl (Dulcolax) is a diphenolic laxative with a chemical structure similar to phenolphthalein. It is absorbed from the gut and deacetylated in the liver to bisacodyl diphenol, which is, in turn, conjugated and excreted in the bile. As in the case of phenolphthalein, the secretion of ingested bisacodyl diphenol in the bile seems necessary for its cathartic action. However, bisacodyl suppositories are rapidly effective upon contact.

Bisacodyl stimulates colon peristalsis and occasional mass movements, which are inhibited if the mucosa is pretreated with local anesthetic. Rectal instillation stimulates the left colon, whereas cecal application initiates a whole colon response. Constipated patients with slow transit usually respond to the drug by rigorous sigmoid contractions. Patients who fail to respond may have damaged myenteric nerves (Chapter 16).

Bisacodyl inhibits water, sodium, and glucose absorption in the small bowel. At one time, it was thought that the net water secretion was due to damage to the mucosa, but it now appears that bisacodyl stimulates adenyl cyclase, an enzyme in mucosal cells which affects cellular secretion through prostaglandin E_2 to cause net intragut water accumulation.

Bisacodyl is commonly used for the treatment of constipation or preparation of the colon for radiographic or endoscopic examination. Peristalsis is initiated in most constipated patients by rectal application of bisacodyl. However, it is doubtful whether any drug with stimulant, irritant, and intracellular effects should be used over long periods. The suppositories may be useful in a bowel-training program, which attempts to wean a patient from laxatives.

The drug is supplied as 5-milligram enteric-coated tablets, or 10-milligram suppositories. Two or three tablets taken by mouth produce soft, formed stools in 6 to 12 hours. The suppository acts in 15 to 20 minutes. Bisacodyl tablets and suppositories are reliable in the preparation of colons for diagnostic procedures. A common regimen is 2 tablets the night before and a suppository the morning of the procedure.

Side effects with bisacodyl are few if the recommended dose is employed. Administration with alkali may allow dissolution of the protective coating of the pills and cause gastric cramps. Most ill effects result from overuse (see below). Bisacodyl and its diphenol may be detected in the urine by liquid chromatography.

Anthracene Glycosides

What rhubarb, senna or what purgative drug,
Would drive these English hence?

Shakespeare, *Macbeth* (5. 3) (or was it Charles de Gaulle?)

Senna and Cascara

Senna and cascara are anthracine glycosides that are more potent on a molar basis than phenolphthalein. These glycosides, like the diphenolic drugs, require colon bacteria to release the active principle. The intact molecule is ineffective when applied directly on the colon. When administered orally, the glycoside is hydrolyzed by the colon flora to release glucose and *aglycones*, the latter being responsible for the laxative effect. However, the aglycones are ineffective when administered orally, apparently requiring the attached sugar to ensure survival through the small gut. Senna acts on the intramural nerve plexes, resulting in decreased sigmoid segmental contractions and increased left colon peristalsis. This local action may be blocked by prior application of a local anesthetic. It is probable that, like many other laxatives, the anthraquinones act on the gut to produce net secretion of water and electrolytes. In rats, a senna preparation (Senokot) decreases jejunum and colon water absorption. This action occurs with neither mucosal damage nor effect on the adenyl cyclase system.

Orally administered, senna and cascara act in 6 to 8 hours. Much is made of their ability to achieve "natural" bowel movements. This notion is based on studies which demonstrate that senna-inspired defecation occurs when spontaneous movements should occur; that is, after meals or exercise. Furthermore, these drugs act on the distal colon producing a solid stool, not a liquid one that might result from a more proximally acting laxative. Such ideal laxation is suggested as part of a bowel-retraining program whereby the drug is gradually replaced by good food and exercise. It is doubtful if a laxative that stimulates and then damages the nerve plexes in the gut can be considered natural (see section on laxative abuse below).

Other Anthracine Glycosides

Frangula, aloes, and rhubarb are found in many patent medicines. Danthron is a sugar-free anthraquinone that is readily absorbed and may turn the urine pink or yellow. Nursing mothers who take this drug may induce diarrhea in their infants. These other anthracine glycosides have been less subject to scientific scrutiny than senna and cascara. Nevertheless, they remain very popular in patent medicines.

Dioctyl Sodium Sulfosuccinate

Widely advertised as a "stool softener," dioctyl sodium sulfosuccinate (DSS) is popularly used to ease defecation following anal surgery. It is a detergent, or "wetting agent," and the stool-softening concept was apparently inspired by a magazine portrayal of a duck, floating on a pond, which sank when DSS was added to the water. However, bile salts and long chain fatty acids are also detergents, and it appears that, like them, DSS alters mucosal water and electrolyte transport. Prostaglandins and cyclic adenosine monophosphate (cyclic-AMP) may mediate this alteration. Therefore, there is no reason to consider it different from the other chemical laxatives. DSS disrupts the epithelium of the stomach and jejunum, and it is said to favor absorption of dyes and mineral oil.

Castor Oil

A most efficacious remedy for the dry bellyach and iliak passion. . . . Castor oil is an excellent cathartic in dysentry; sheathing the intestines from acrimony and irritation and well adapted to relieve tortima and tenesmus.

James Thatcher (1821)

Castor oil, a triglyceride extracted from the seeds of tropical plants, has been used as a cathartic for 3,500 years. The word *castor* as applied to the oil apparently comes from a Jamaican plant that is believed to reduce sexual appetite. Certainly, nobody would accuse castor oil of being an aphrodisiac. The triglyceride is hydrolyzed in the small gut by enzymes to release glycerol and ricinoleic acid, with the latter stimulating gut motility and intraluminal fluid and electrolyte accumulation.

Ricinoleate, the active metabolite of castor oil, causes net secretion of water, sodium, and chloride, and a state of altered mucosal permeability. Unlike the effect of cholera enterotoxin, this altered permeability is due to damage to the colon and small intestinal mucosa. Animal studies suggest roles for prostaglandin E_2, cyclic AMP, and certain mucosal enzymes, but the altered permeability could result from the mucosal damage.

This powerful drug apparently has an effect by other than the oral route. The use of a mixture of the oil with calamine on babies' bottoms results in diarrhea. Early military aircraft used castor oil as a lubricant, so that the Red Baron was not the only reason why World War I pilots made frequent returns to base. Oral administration of castor oil produces abdominal cramps and loose bowel movements within 2 hours. Although it has been advocated in the treatment of worms, less toxic laxatives are available. Because of its high affinity for drugs used in psychiatric disorders, it has been employed in the treatment of overdose. Otherwise, castor oil has little, if any, place in modern medicine.

OSMOTIC LAXATIVES

Saline Cathartics

Since medieval times, organic salts have been employed as purgatives. Evidently, such treatment was available in the fourteenth century at the Carlsbad spa. When, in 1618, it was noted that the oxen of Henry Wicks refused the bitter waters of Epsom, a new patent medicine was born. The saline laxatives are magnesium and sodium salts. Magnesium and sulfate are the active ions (phosphate and tartrate to a lesser extent). The salines have long been thought to hold water in the lumen by osmosis and thus induce laxation by increasing the water delivered to the colon. Some researchers have advanced the hypothesis that magnesium and other ions act by releasing cholecystokinin (CCK) from the duodenum. Like CCK, saline purgatives increase small-bowel and colon motility and stimulate pancreatic, bile, and small-bowel secretion of fluid.

Magnesium sulfate (epsom salts) is bitter and unpleasant tasting. A semifluid evacuation occurs less than 3 hours after a dose of 5 to 15 grams. Therefore, it is used to rid the gut of blood in patients with liver failure, of drugs in poisonings, and of worms after the administration of a vermifuge. Milk of magnesia (magnesium hydroxide), an essential ingredient of most antacid preparations, is a milder saline laxative.

Salts containing magnesium are a potential hazard to those with impaired kidney function, since up to 25 percent may be ab-

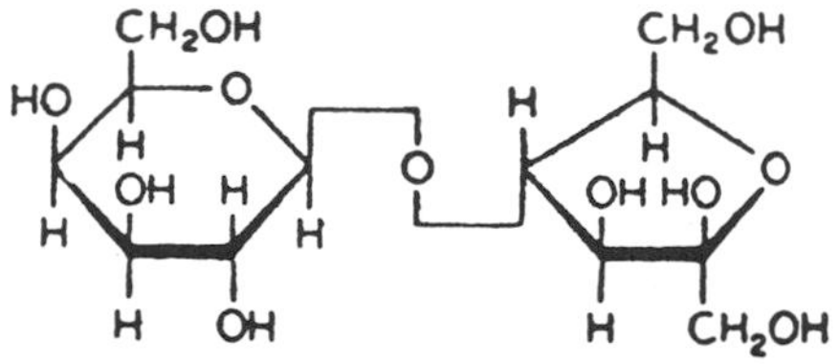

Figure 28. Lactulose is a disaccharide consisting of two molecules of the monosaccharide galactose joined by an oxygen bond. Since this bond cannot be split by intestinal mucosal enzymes as in the case of other disaccharides (eg, lactose, sucrose), the lactulose arrives in the colon intact. There it is destroyed by bacteria, releasing hydrogen and osmotically active products. The fate of lactulose is similar to that of lactose in persons without the mucosal enzyme lactase (see Figure 19).

sorbed. Sodium sulfate or phosphate may be used orally or as an enema, provided sodium retention is not a concern as in heart failure (see also the section on Enemas below).

Lactulose

Lactulose is a disaccharide consisting of 2 galactose molecules joined by an oxygen bond (Figure 28). Although it resembles lactose in structure, lactulose has no corresponding disaccharidase on human intestinal mucosal cells (see Chapter 11). Thus, digestion and absorption fail to occur in the small intestine, and lactulose reaches the colon intact. In the ascending colon, lactulose is degraded by the local gut flora within 20 to 30 minutes, producing lactic and acetic acid.

Lactulose acidifies the stool and reduces the raised blood ammonia found in patients with liver failure. However, it is the cathartic effects of lactulose that concern us here. The diarrheogenic effect appears to result from the osmotic action of unabsorbed sugar. Lactulose increases stool weight, volume, and water content. In a double-blind study of constipated laxative users, 80 percent improved on lactulose when other drugs were discontinued compared to 33 percent on placebo. The drug is also suitable for children and is as effective as senna but with fewer side effects.

Lactulose syrup appears to be particularly useful in the elderly. In one 12-week double-blind trial, 47 elderly residents of a nursing home were treated with 30 grams of either glucose or lactulose. Compared to glucose, those receiving lactulose had less fecal impaction, required fewer enemas, and had less cramps, bloating, flatulence, and tenesmus. Another controlled study produced similar results and further demonstrated that lactulose reduced the nursing time required in the care of elderly incompetent patients, many of whom were on constipating medication.

The usual adult dose of lactulose for constipation is 15 milliliters daily (1 tablespoonful), which may be increased until the desired effect is achieved. Although many users complain of the sweet taste, lactulose is well tolerated by the elderly. The drug is nontoxic and the only important side effect is hypokalemia, which one might expect from any diarrhea. If one must use a laxative other than a bulk-former, lactulose has a lot to recommend it.

OBSOLETE LAXATIVES

A number of traditional laxatives, or *drastics*, are downright dangerous.

Mercurous Chloride

As recently as 1974, two poisonings and one death resulted from a mercury cathartic. The dead person had for 20 years consumed each night a tablet containing 120 milligrams of mercurous chloride. Near death, the patient had blue sclera and suffered intractable diarrhea, renal failure, and dementia. Of particular interest at autopsy was the presence of a white pseudomembrane overlying the colon mucosa. Mercurous chloride, which is contained in calomel and "blue pill," was extensively used in the nineteenth century. Reports of 100 years ago of what has been interpreted as the IBS laid great stress on the presence of a pseudomembrane, which might be passed as a perfect cast of the bowel. Since we seldom observe this phenomenon today, could these pseudomembranes have resulted from the use of such toxic cathartics as mercury?

Other Obsolete Purgatives

Croton oil is a mucosal irritant that was used in bygone days to alter the political views of prisoners. It is one of the most violent of all purgatives. When applied to the skin, it induces blisters, and a single drop in the mouth causes vomiting, colic, and extreme diarrhea. Obviously, such treatment is not for the timid. Podophyllin, a cytotoxic resin used to remove warts, cannot be considered a practical cathartic, but it still exists in some over-the-counter laxative mixtures. Oral bile salts directly stimulate the colon and inhibit the absorption of salt and water. The resultant catharsis explains the durability of a patent medicine called Caroid and Bile Salts. Because of adverse effects on the gastric mucosa, this ancient preparation should not be used. Along with strychnine, jalap, and colocynth, these drugs have no place in any medicine chest.

PER RECTUM EVACUANTS

Suppositories

The ancient physicians of Egypt, Greece, and Rome used the rectum as a port for medication, and the apothecaries in the middle ages prepared medicated balls of honey for rectal insertion. In the eighteenth century, cocoa butter was discovered. Because this product remains firm at room temperature, yet melts with body heat, it proved to be an ideal base for a suppository.

Glycerine suppositories contain about 70 percent glycerine, sometimes with added sodium stearate (a fatty acid). Because of its lubricating and hydroscopic action when inserted, a glycerine suppository stimulates the defecation reflex. This suppository thus

Table 29
Per Rectum Evacuants

Suppositories
  Glycerine
  Bisacodyl
Enemas
  Lactulose (for liver failure)
  Tap water
  Saline
  Soapsuds (obsolete)
  Retention
    Olive oil
    Arachis oil
  Disposable
    Sodium phosphate
    Biphosphate (Fleet)

seems harmless and may be useful in a bowel-training program in which pharmacological stimulation is undesirable (Table 29).

Acting directly and reflexly on the large bowel, a bisacodyl suppository should produce a bowel movement in 15 to 20 minutes. The suppository should not be buried in the stool as little effect will ensue. It is also of elementary as well as eliminatory importance to remove the wrapper of the suppository. A few individuals who use suppositories may experience rectal irritation, or possibly damage to the rectal mucosa.

Enemas

One of the essential gifts one should look for in a wife is the ability to administer an enema daily and pleasantly.

Voltaire (1694–1778)

Like suppositories, enemas have been handed down from antiquity. They once graced the court of King Louis XIV, when enema stools were as common as footstools in the parlors of France. Early in this century, when colon contents were believed the source of many illnesses, enemas were encouraged. In London, there were "colon laundries" set up for this purpose. Currently, the enema is in relative decline, although it still has its uses.

Some medications, for example, can be introduced into patients by enema. Lactulose or neomycin enemas are employed in patients with coma that is due to liver failure. Hydrocortisone and 5-aminosalicylic acid enemas are useful in ulcerative colitis. But the most prevalent use of enemas is to evacuate the colon in constipated patients or in those preparing for surgery, barium enema, or colonoscopy.

It is believed by many doctors and nurses that irrigation of the whole colon by up to 8 liters of warm fluid results in a cleansing effect. It is also stated that the sole justification for an enema is to stimulate the rectum by distension. The embarrassing truth is that we do not know much more about how enemas work than did King Louis himself. Tap water enemas are popular, but isotonic saline minimizes fluid and electrolyte shifts. Saline should be used cautiously in heart or kidney failure.

Oil Retention Enemas

In patients with fecal impaction, rectal injection of 100 cubic centimeters of olive or peanut oil may soften the feces so that a small saline enema might subsequently be successful. Impacted stool distends the anal sphincter, interfering with the defecation reflex. A crammed anal canal makes insertion of an enema tip risky. Under these circumstances, there is no alternative for the physician or nurse but to roll up his sleeves, don rubber gloves, and disimpact the rectum manually.

Disposable Enemas

A compound prepared from sodium phosphate-biphosphate is commercially available in a small single-dose plastic container (Fleet enema, Fletcher's enema) and is typically promoted as a "disposable enema." (Are there any enemas that one would save?) This hyperosmolar saline cathartic is useful in fecal and barium impaction and cleanses satisfactorily the left colon for fiberoptic sigmoidoscopy (Chapter 22). By attracting water into the lumen, the enema expands and wets the stool.

Whole Gut Irrigation

Several liters of fluid administered orally over 2 to 3 hours can prepare the colon for surgery. Bowel movements commence in 40 to 60 minutes and become clear by 90 minutes. Those patients who are liable to heart failure may require a diuretic. In a randomized trial in 75 patients, this irrigation technique appeared to be almost as successful in preparing colons for barium enemas as a 3-day procedure consisting of low-residue diet, castor oil, and enemas. Most patients prefer the lavage, and it is the treatment of choice in many units.

A current regimen is as follows: A 4-liter plastic bottle containing polyethylene glycol, sodium chloride, potassium chloride, sodium bicarbonate, and sodium sulfate is filled with water to thoroughly mix the salts. After a 3-hour fast, the subject drinks 240 milliliters (8 ounces) every 6 minutes until the fecal discharge is clear. Three to 4 liters are usually required.

MELANOSIS COLI

Melanosis coli is a sign of chronic laxative use. In this condition, the normally pink, glistening rectal mucosa is stained dark brown or mahogany, with the design being homogeneous, mottled, or patchy. Frequently, it is two-toned, with dark geometric spots appearing as paving stones with an interlacing yellow background. To some observers it resembles nutmeg, whereas others liken it to toad, snake, crocodile, or tiger skin. The peculiar color is due to a melaninlike pigment of unknown origin beneath the colon mucosa. Curiously, the pigmentation ends abruptly at the ileocecal valve.

In 1931, melanosis coli was discovered in 11 percent of colons at autopsy, 17 percent in those over 40. In a series of 553 sigmoidoscopies done in 1933, melanosis was present in 4.7 percent, but it seems to be less prevalent today. For example, in 200 consecutive examinations, we did not see a single case. Occasionally, the pigment may be detected only microscopically. The discoloration usually appears a year or more after commencing anthraquinone laxatives such as senna, cascara, or danthron, and it fades away several months after they are discontinued. Such pigmentation does not occur with the use of osmotic or diphenolic laxatives, but its discovery does provide incontrovertible evidence of chronic anthraquinone abuse.

LAXATIVE ABUSE

Nearly all men die of their medicines, not of their diseases.

Molière (1622–1673), *La Maladie Imaginaire*

As to prevent our maladies unseen,
We sicken to shun sickness when we purge.

Shakespeare, Sonnet 118

The folly of self-medication was certainly recognized in the golden age of literature, but regrettably, in this golden age of medicine and public enlightenment, such folly endures. Twenty-four percent of 254 consecutive patients used laxatives regularly and 10 percent abused these products. Twenty-two percent of 301 apparently healthy British adults used laxatives, 6 percent more often than twice a week. In the United States, 3.4 percent of young people use laxatives at least once a month. It is difficult to understand those few individuals who complain of diarrhea and yet hide their laxative use from their doctors. In one report, 27 patients with chronic diarrhea were referred after extensive investigations to a tertiary care hospital in Texas. There, it was found that 7 patients were secretly taking laxatives and 2 were taking diuretics. Another report described 17 surreptitious laxative users, of whom 16 were discovered by stool tests and one was exposed by room search. Most laxative abusers are women. Some practice bulemia for which binge eating is atoned by self-induced vomiting, purging, or diuresis. The cost of this practice is self-evident, and the consequences can very often be life-threatening.

Chronic administration of anthracine cathartics can cause damage in the myenteric nerves in the colons of mice and men. Thus an individual may become physiologically as well as psychologically dependent on catharsis, since the colon fails to work without its laxative fix. Drastic purgation may produce a diarrhea so severe that water and sodium depletion results. In such a condition, subsequent release by the kidney of the hormones renin and aldosterone leads, in turn, to potassium loss.

Studies have shown that malabsorption and intestinal protein loss may occur as well in laxative abuse. Two patients are reported to have had finger clubbing as a result of senna abuse. In one of these cases, the clubbing disappeared when the senna was withdrawn, only to reappear when the glycoside was resumed. Hypocalcemic tetany (muscle spasm) may also result from the injudicious use of hypertonic phosphate enemas.

In keeping with myenteric nerve damage, there is a characteristic radiographic picture of cathartic colon. The loss of haustra and smooth, tapering pseudostrictures may be mistaken for colitis (Figure 29). It is by no means certain, however, that the radiographic picture is due simply to the laxatives. Recognition of primary pseudo-obstruction syndromes gives the physician cause to wonder which is primary—the atonic colon or the laxative abuse?

Diagnosis of Laxative Abuse

There is seldom a satisfactory explanation for a patient's concealment of his or her laxative use while investigation of diarrhea is in progress. Most such patients are women and many are connected to medicine in some way. Common manifestations include diarrhea, although some individuals may claim to be constipated,

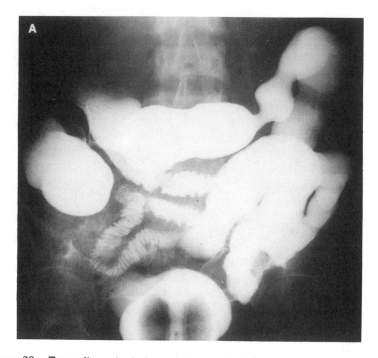

Figure 29. Two radiographs during a single examination of a 72-year-old woman with cathartic colon who for 25 to 30 years had daily ingested a tablet containing aloin, senna, cascara, and belladonna. A barium enema done 4 years previously had reportedly shown ulcerative colitis. A sigmoidoscopy showed melanosis coli. Withdrawal of the laxative and daily bran ingestion resulted in a satisfactory bowel habit, but the colon x-ray was unchanged 6 months later. (A) Note the loss of normal colon haustra, as compared with Figure 26. Narrowing, which is transient, can be seen in the ascending colon and splenic flexure. (B) The pseudostrictures are now distended with barium. Although there are no ulcers, and the colon is not foreshortened, the appearances were originally interpreted as those of ulcerative colitis.   (continued on page 302)

with weakness, vague aches and pains, and emotional lability. A "locker search" is the time-honored way to expose the laxative habits of these misguided patients. Otherwise, the physician's only recourse may be analysis of stool or urine for laxative traces. The easiest to detect is phenolphthalein, the conjugate of which may

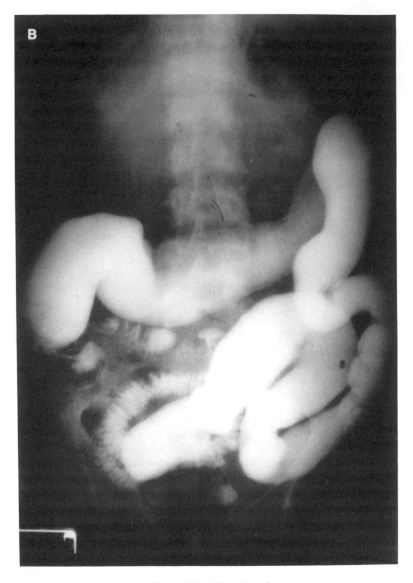

Figure 29.   (*Continued*)

be excreted in the urine for several days after a single dose. In the laboratory, the drug must be deconjugated by boiling the urine with sodium hydroxide. If phenolphthalein is present, it will turn red. Stool containing phenolpthalein may also blush with alkalinization. Bisacodyl and its diphenol may be detected in urine by gas–liquid chromatography; and there are specific assays for anthraquinone derivatives as well. A sigmoidoscopic appearance of melanosis coli is strong evidence of anthraquinone use. A stool phosphate content of greater than 4.5 milliquivalents per liter suggests phosphate use. In the study of 17 laxative abusers, one was confirmed by locker search, and the remainder by stool analysis.

Treatment

It is one thing to prove that a patient's diarrhea is due to laxative abuse; it may be quite another matter to alter the situation. If the damage to the colon is reversible, than recovery may follow introduction of bulking agents and the cessation of cathartics. Alas, "there's the rub": for many such patients simply will not stop, or stop denying, laxative abuse.

Excessive use of cathartics is not confined to eccentric patients. Fifty years ago, an Oxford professor of medicine, L. J. Witts, urged his colleagues to refrain from ritual purgation. He pointed out that preoperative purging of "any unfortunate patient who is robust enough to stand the strain" is a practice "rooted in archaic and primitive beliefs rather than physiology and pathology."

ENEMA ABUSE

Lack of care in the placement of an enema tip can result in a perforated rectum. In 32 such disasters, the patients were very ill; 8 died, and 4 required a permanent colostomy. Particularly nasty perforations result from the careless insertions of "disposable" enema tips. Hypertonic phosphate in the tissues is very destructive and may necessitate a colostomy. There is evidence that the resulting inflammation might be improved by prednisone. The traditional soapsuds enema should be a thing of the past. In the grim halflight of the evening shift, enema duty frequently falls to the most junior nurse, who might be forgiven for believing that if a little soap is good, a lot is better. Thus, the 5 percent soap formula may easily be exceeded. Further, soap containing fatty acids may deliver large quantities of sodium. Soap enemas have caused anaphylaxis, colitis with shock that is due to fluid loss, and heart muscle depression that is due to hypokalemia. The following case illustrates the devastating effects of the wanton use of soap enemas:

> A 55-year-old woman with alcoholic cirrhosis was admitted in liver coma with a very low serum potassium. Her husband explained that he had administered soapsuds enemas daily for two months in order to "get rid of the ammonia." A large dose of intravenous potassium chloride was necessary before the serum potassium was restored to normal and the coma reversed.

SUMMARY

The regular use of dietary fiber is the most physiologic and effective means of preventing constipation. In those individuals who find a high-fiber diet difficult, bran or psyllium may be employed. Because of the risk of lipoid pneumonia and also of fat-soluble vitamin malabsorption, mineral oil use has no place in modern medicine. Dioctyl sodium sulfosuccinate is not a special kind of stool softener but rather is a "stimulant" laxative like senna or cascara. Following surgery, or in preparation for a procedure, senna or bisacodyl may be used. Rapidly acting osmotic agents, such as magnesium sulfate, are useful in the treatment of liver coma that is due to blood in the gut, or of intestinal worms, in which quick results are desired. Lactulose, the osmotic laxative, is effective in the treatment of liver coma, and this sweet syrup is particularly popular with constipated children or seniors. Of the per rectum evacuants, suppositories have a mainly mechanical action, although bisacodyl topically stimulates the colon. Isotonic saline enemas are sometimes required in the preparation for a procedure, for evacuation following surgery, or as part of a bowel-retraining program. Oil-retention enemas may soften the stool in patients with fecal impaction but should not be used as an excuse to delay manual disimpaction. Phosphate disposable enemas, if given with care, provide a safe, quick evacuation.

The principal significance of laxatives in gut reactions results from their abuse. Chronic employment of stimulant laxatives may result in an unresponsive, atonic colon and intransigent constipation. Patients who are using anthraquinone laxatives may be found to have melanosis coli. Careless use of any colon cleanout procedure may deplete the patient of sodium, water, and potassium. Diarrhea patients who self-medicate themselves with large doses of laxatives, even when they admit it, may be very difficult to manage.

CHAPTER TWENTY

Drugs and the Irritable Gut

Doctors are men who prescribe medicine of which they know little to cure diseases of which they know less in human beings of which they know nothing.

Voltaire (1694–1778)

Many drugs have been tried with little success in the syndromes of the irritable gut. Yet, despite this lack of benefit, some gut reactions to drugs are undoubted. In the previous chapter, we saw that laxatives can do more harm than good in chronic functional syndromes. In this chapter, we will be concerned with the gut effects of drugs that are used for nongut illnesses. Upon perusal of drug formularies, it appears that few drugs fail to have potential gut side effects. Much suffering might be avoided if the constipated patient with back pain would discontinue codeine, or if the diarrhea patient with peptic ulcers would restrict the use of magnesium-containing antacids. Such undesirable effects are so ubiquitous that, on principle, any drug that the gut complainant takes should be suspect.

It is impractical to catalog all the side effects that are known or suspected or that are understood or not understood. Therefore, in this chapter, we will concentrate on those classes of drugs that

Table 30
Gut Side Effects of Some Classes of Drugs

	Nausea, vomiting	Diarrhea	Constipation	Abdominal pain
Cholinergic (bethanecol)	+	+		+
Cholinesterase inhibitors (Tensilon, Mestinon)	+	+		+
Anticholinergic M₁, M₂ antagonists (tricyclics, phenothiazines)			+	
M₁ antagonist (pirenzepine)		+		
Adrenergic α₂ agonist (clonidine, lidamadine)			+	
Antiadrenergic α₁ antagonist (phentolamine)	+	+		+
β₁, β₂ antagonists (propranolol)	+	+		+
Dopamine D₁, D₂ agonists (L-dopa, bromocriptine)	+		+	+
Opiates			+	
⁺⁺Ca channel blockers			+	
Prostaglandins		+		+
Erythromycin	+			+

have gut receptors known to transmit pharmacologic effects (Table 30). In the interest of a more complete explanation of gut effects, drugs within these classes that are used for gastrointestinal complaints will be included as examples. An understanding of these should help the reader predict undesirable drug effects. Many drugs that are said, without authority, to cause gut symptoms will be omitted.

CHOLINERGICS AND ANTICHOLINERGICS

Acetylcholine is a neurotransmitter substance that excites enteric nerves and gut smooth muscle. It is generally associated with the vagus and other parasympathetic nerves. The muscle has *muscarinic* receptors, and the nerve synapses (junctions) have *nicotinic* receptors. Two types of muscarinic receptors, M_1 and M_2, mediate different effects in different tissues. Cholinergic nerves enhance intestinal smooth muscle tone and motility, relax sphincters, and thereby ease the passage of chyme through the gut. The cholinergic drugs, methacholine (Mecholyl) and bethanechol (Urecholine), are potent cholinergic receptor stimulants, the latter being used to treat a lazy bladder or urinary retention. Bethanechol provides more stimulation to the gut than to other tissues, and, unlike acetylcholine, is resistant to inactivation by the natural enzyme cholinesterase. It causes both small-bowel and colon contractions that produce colicky abdominal pain, nausea, and diarrhea. Some patients with gastroesophageal reflux improve when cholinergic drugs are used to augment peristalsis and to increase lower esophageal sphincter tone.

Cholinesterase inhibitors increase acetylcholine survival at nerve and muscle receptors, thus prolonging cholinergic effects. Such drugs are used for the paralyzing disease myasthenia gravis. Examples include neostigmine (Prostigmin), edrophonium (Tensilon), and pyridostigmine (Mestinon). The cholinergic symptoms of nausea, vomiting, cramps, and diarrhea may occur with their use. In fact, edrophonium's ability to cause gut smooth muscle contraction has led to its use for the provocation of esophageal spasm during motility studies of patients with noncardiac chest pain (Chapter 9).

Atropine is an important drug that blocks cholinergic receptors on the gut. This natural anticholinergic inhibits the motor activity of the stomach, small bowel, and colon. Atropine and other anticholinergic drugs, such as dicyclomine (Bentylol, Bentyl), inhibit the meal-induced, cholinergic gastrocolonic response; that is, increased colon myoelectric and motor activity. This is the rationale (as yet unproven) for their use in IBS patients with meal-induced pain. Because the commonly used phenothiazine tranquilizers and tricyclic antidepressants have anticholinergic properties, constipation frequently occurs with the use of these drugs. Similar drugs that are used for Parkinson's disease also have anticholinergic effects.

Cholinergic drugs induce net secretion in the small intestine by reducing water and chloride absorption. These effects are also inhibited by the anticholinergic atropine. Thus, drugs with cholinergic effects through stimulation of gut activity cause nausea, vomiting, diarrhea, and abdominal cramps. Anticholinergics have the opposite effects. However, cholinergic receptors are very complex, and researchers strive to develop drugs that maximize beneficial effects and minimize the detrimental ones. Such a drug is pirenzepine (Gastrozepin), which blocks M_1 receptors and suppresses gastric secretion with less anticholinergic effect elsewhere.

Adrenergics and Antiadrenergics

The sympathetic nervous system regulates many organs including the gastrointestinal tract. Sympathetic stimulation is mediated by the natural neurotransmitter norepinephrine. Drugs that partly or completely mimic norepinephrine are called *adrenergic*. Like the cholinergic receptors, the adrenergic receptors are very complex. The development of more specific adrenergic agents permits greater understanding of adrenergic effects on gastrointestinal motility. Sympathetic nerves appear to regulate cholinergic enteric nerves, modifying the contractile state of the gut. Four types of adrenergics are identified: α_1 and α_2 receptors and β_1 and β_2 receptors.

Alpha receptor stimulation relaxes colon muscle. The antihypertensive drug clonidine (Catapres) stimulates α_1 receptors to delay gastrointestinal transit, and may produce constipation at doses used to treat hypertension. Some of clonidine's constipating effect is due to the stimulation of alpha receptors in the gut mucosa, which promote water absorption. Lidamidine, an experimental alpha-stimulating drug developed from clonidine, is an antidiarrheal agent.

Adrenergic nervous activity has been demonstrated to suppress gastrointestinal motility after abdominal surgery. In a study of such patients the beta-blocking drug propranolol (Inderal) induced intestinal recovery more quickly than a placebo. In another group of postoperative patients, dihydroergotamine (an α_1 blocker) produced the first bowel movement sooner than placebo.

Propranolol, which blocks both β_1 and β_2 receptors, increases peristalsis in the distal esophagus and lower esophageal sphincter (LES) and shortens gastric emptying time. Theoretically, it might help heartburn and worsen esophageal spasm. Intravenous propranolol increases colon contractions in patients with IBS and produces symptoms in some of these patients. The β_1 blocker metaprolol (Lopressor) increases colon motility in healthy volunteers at doses used for hypertension or angina.

In summary, alpha agonists, alpha antagonists, and beta blockers, which are used in the treatment of heart disease and hypertension, have a variety of gut effects. Such α_2 stimulants as clonidine may constipate, whereas the α_1 antagonists such as phentolamine (Regitine) may cause nausea, vomiting, and abdominal cramps. Similar symptoms occur with beta blockers and constitute the most frequent side effects of these commonly used drugs.

Dopaminergic and Antidopaminergic Agents

Dopamine inhibits stomach contractions and blocks coordination of the stomach and the duodenum. Apparently, there are 2 dopaminergic receptors, D_1 and D_2. Domperidone (Motilium) is a D_2 dopamine antagonist that reverses these gastric effects. In patients with diabetic gastric paralysis, domperidone and metoclopramide (Maxeran) improve gastric emptying. Some metoclopramide effect may be blocked by atropine, suggesting a partial cholinergic mechanism.

About 80 percent of patients treated for Parkinson's disease with the dopaminergic drug levodopa (L-dopa) experience loss of appetite, nausea, vomiting, epigastric discomfort, and constipation. These effects are partially transmitted through the vomiting center in the brain, but mainly through dopamine receptors in the gut. Another drug used in Parkinson's disease, bromocriptine (Parlodel), exerts similar dopaminergic effects on the gut. These adverse drug reactions may be alleviated by the D_2 antagonist domperidone without reducing the antiparkinsonian effect. Other antinausea and vomiting effects of dopamine antagonists are mediated through the brain.

Dopamine also increases nonpropulsive colon contractions. This may explain the constipation induced by antiparkinsonian drugs. Domperidone inhibits these contractions, but does not change motor activity of the sigmoid colon in patients with IBS. Thus, the dopaminergic drugs levodopa and bromocriptine cause nausea, vomiting, and constipation, which may be prevented by the D_2 antagonist domperidone.

OPIATES AND OPIATE ANTAGONISTS

Morphine, an alkaloid of opium, was used for diarrhea before it was used as a pain reliever. Opiate receptors are present in the central nervous system, in peripheral nerves, and throughout the gastrointestinal tract. There appear to be three opiate receptors: mu, delta, and kappa. The relative importance of these receptors is uncertain, but the different effects of various opiates on gut function apparently depend upon which receptors they stimulate.

Intravenously, morphine lowers LES pressure and delays gastric emptying. Opiates also prolong total bowel transit time by increasing intestinal tone and segmental nonperistaltic colon contractions, effects that impair propulsion. Thus, morphine constipates by delayed gastric emptying, reduced small and large bowel transit, increased anal sphincter tone, and inattention to the urge to defecate. With continuous use of opiates, some tolerance develops.

The mechanisms by which other opiates produce constipation are similar in nature but different in degree. Synthetic narcotics, such as pentazocine (Talwin) and meperidine (Demerol), produce less constipation than morphine at equivalent pain-killing doses.

The effects of opiates on gastrointestinal motility are mediated directly and also via the brain and spinal cord. Etorphine acts mainly at the central level, methadone (Amidone) acts centrally and peripherally, and morphine acts mainly peripherally. Less morphine is required to affect gut motility than to relieve pain. Some antidiarrheal effect may be due to the inhibition of mucosal secretion.

There are also natural or endogenous opiates in the body that have both analgesic (pain-relieving) and gut motility effects. The small intestine contains an abundance of *enkephalins*, mainly in the myenteric ganglia and smooth muscle. The opiate antagonist naloxone (Narcan) increases fecal weight and frequency in elderly patients with constipation. Since naloxone is poorly absorbed, it must exert its effects directly on the gut. This implies that endogenous opiates affect gastrointestinal motility, and may help explain such drug effects as the placebo response (Chapter 21).

In summary, narcotics delay gastric emptying, slow transit time, and perhaps reduce gut secretion. In some people and also with some doses of narcotic agents, nausea, vomiting, loss of appetite, and constipation may occur. Loperamide (Imodium), diphenoxylate (Lomotil), and codeine act peripherally and are used as antidiarrheal agents (Chapter 15). Loperamide is the favored antidiarrheal opiate because it fails to penetrate the central nervous system.

CALCIUM CHANNEL BLOCKERS

The influx of calcium ions into smooth muscle cells generates the electrical activity that results in muscle contraction. This influx occurs through calcium channels in the cell membrane. The calcium channel blockers are a class of drugs that are used mainly for cardiac disorders. They also relax the smooth muscle of small arteries and are therefore used in hypertension and in the vascular spasm found in Raynaud's phenomenon. They have been tried with limited success in the "nutcracker" esophagus (Chapter 9).

Calcium channel blockers that are used in coronary artery disease, especially verapamil (Isoptin), cause constipation. Intravenous calcium chloride may relieve constipation and fecal impaction caused by verapamil, but it is not a practical antidote. Some of the antidiarrheal effects of loperamide may be mediated through calcium channel antagonism.

In IBS patients, sublingual nifedipine (Adalat) reduces the gastrocolonic response; however, there are no studies showing clinical benefit in the IBS. Considering the poor correlation between gut symptoms and gut motor and electrical activity, it cannot be predicted that calcium channel blockers will be useful in the IBS or in diarrhea. Nonetheless, these drugs may be expected to constipate when used for nongut disorders.

PROSTAGLANDINS

Prostaglandins are distributed widely in the mucosa and muscle of the gastrointestinal tract. They act directly on the smooth muscle and indirectly via nerve receptors. The effects of prostaglandins on intestinal motility depend upon the type of prostaglandin, its concentration, and even the muscle studied. Some prostaglandins alter gastrointestinal secretion by inhibiting sodium absorption and increasing chloride and water secretion in the small bowel. These effects and the reduced colon transit time can result in diarrhea.

Prostaglandins (prostin E_2) that are used therapeutically to induce or maintain uterine contractions during labor, frequently cause diarrhea. The antiulcer prostaglandin, misoprostil (Cytotec), also causes diarrhea. Such laxatives as ricinoleic acid (castor oil), oleic acid, bisacodyl, and phenolphthalein stimulate intestinal prostaglandin synthesis (Chapter 19).

ANTIBIOTICS

Diarrhea may accompany treatment with any antibiotic and seems to be caused by several mechanisms. Diarrhea commonly occurs with ampicillin and probably results from altered colon flora. Pseudomembranous colitis is a severe acute disorder that is due to antibiotic-facilitated overgrowth of *Clostridium difficile*, a cytotoxin-producing bacterium. Unlike a simple antibiotic-associated diarrhea, pseudomembranous colitis may require hospitalization and antibiotic therapy.

The antibiotic erythromycin commonly causes abdominal pain, nausea, and vomiting and appears to alter directly small-bowel motility.

MISCELLANEOUS DRUGS

The diarrhea that is encountered with some antacid preparations is due to the osmotic effect of magnesium hydroxide. The constipating effect of calcium carbonate and aluminum hydroxide is not so well understood (Chapter 10). Digitalis, which is used for heart disease, causes nausea and vomiting. Both oral colchicine used for gout, and intravenous vasopressin, used to control gastrointestinal bleeding, cause diarrhea. The use of sucralfate for peptic ulcers and cholestyramine for high blood cholesterol may constipate. The antirheumatic, nonsteroidal analgesics that are represented by aspirin and indomethacin (Indocin) cause stomach ulcers and dyspepsia. The list of unwanted gut effects of drugs is seemingly endless and the mechanisms are often unknown. Any gut symptom must lead the physician to suspect any drug that the sufferer is currently taking.

On the other hand, many putative side effects of drugs are not clearly established. Placebo-controlled trials have taught us that placebos can induce gut symptoms (see Chapter 21). Thus, minor gut complaints of a patient on essential drugs must be evaluated carefully before the drug is withdrawn.

SUMMARY

Recognition of specific receptors in the enteric nervous system has permitted us to begin to understand the effects of some drugs on the gut. Such knowledge should help us predict how various classes of drugs may act. We have concentrated here on drug

groups that stimulate and block cholinergic, adrenergic, dopaminergic, opiate, prostaglandin, and calcium channel receptors. It is
likely that new receptors and drugs that affect them will eventually
be recognized. For the present, it would be wise to suspect any
drug that the patient has taken as a cause of a new symptom. In
the absence of a logical explanation, the physician should critically
evaluate the new symptom in the light of known pharmacology,
and also consider the imponderable side effects that are due to
placebo, which are discussed in the next chapter.

CHAPTER TWENTY-ONE

Clinical Trials and the Placebo Response

The desire to take medicine is one feature which distinguishes man the animal from his fellow creatures. It is really one of the most serious difficulties with which we have to contend. Even with minor ailments . . . the doctor's visit is not thought to be complete without a prescription.

Sir William Osler (1895)

THE NEED FOR CLINICAL TRIALS

When a surgeon lances a boil, the relief is instantaneous, and nobody doubts the efficacy of this procedure. Science is observation. The beneficial effect of penicillin in pneumococcal pneumonia or of appendectomy in acute appendicitis are readily accepted by everyone as effective and even life-saving treatments. In these cases, the illness is acute, the treatment specific, and the end point is obvious to all. Therefore, it may be surprising to learn that most medical (and surgical) treatments are not so easy to validate. Much of what physicians do therapeutically is instinctive, sensible, but without proof of efficacy. Nowhere is this more true than in the treatment of the chronic, recurrent, benign, usually incurable disorders of the irritable gut.

Efficacy of a treatment is easy to prove when the end point (cure or improvement) is rapid and obvious. There should be an objective abnormality, that is, one that may be observed to improve by other than the physician and the patient. In the irritable bowel syndrome (IBS) and other gut reactions, the symptoms are subjective. No one but the sufferer can measure pain, so judgment of improvement relies on his or her say-so. If the symptoms are chronic and recurrent, it may take some weeks or months before the treated person can judge himself improved. The irritable gut sufferer is seldom cured, so judgment of improvement is subject to many biases resulting from individual interpretation, changing attitudes, and what is known as the placebo response. In an attempt to circumvent these difficulties, clinical trials have been developed. Although this technique is now commonplace and is responsible for the validation of many modern treatments, it remains a blunt instrument and has many shortcomings in the irritable gut.

PRINCIPLES OF A CLINICAL TRIAL

The simplest clinical trials are those carried out in a physician's office every day. The patient has a symptom, and the physician tries a drug or diet that is based on his experience and knowledge. If the symptom is improved, everyone is happy, provided the treatment has no harmful effect. Often, the physician cannot prove from the available published evidence that the treatment is generally effective for that symptom. An extension of this is the use of the treatment for a series of patients with the same symptom. Then, if the physician finds that it satisfies most sufferers of the symptom, he gains confidence in the treatment and uses it more often, and sometimes for other symptoms as well. As we shall see, this process, however practical and sensible, is quite unscientific and subject to bias. Otherwise, how could bloodletting, acupuncture, or megavitamins have become so fashionable in their times?

This problem of bias has led to the concept of a controlled

clinical trial. The first scientific foray into this difficult area was performed by James Lind, a British naval surgeon, on board the HMS *Salisbury* in 1747. At that time, many sailors suffered and died of scurvy during long sea voyages. We now know that their diet, which was devoid of fruit and vegetables, lacked vitamin C. Many nostrums were employed at the time without a rational basis, without scientific validation, and certainly without success. In order to discredit the nostrums and convince the navy of the value of fruits, Lind (1953) conducted the following experiment.

> On the 20th of May 1747, I took 12 patients in the scurvy on board the Salisbury at sea. Their cases were as similar as I could have them. They all in general had putrid gums, the spots and lassitude, with weakness of their knees. They lay together in one place, being a proper apartment for the sick in the forehold; and one diet common to all. . . . Two of these were ordered each a quart of cider a day. Two others took 25 gutts of elixir vitriol 3 times a day. . . . Two others took 2 teaspoons of vinegar 3 times a day. . . . Two of the worst patients . . . were put on a course of sea water. . . . Two others had each 2 oranges and 1 lemon given them every day. . . . The two remaining patients took the biggness of a nutmeg 3 times a day, of an electuary recommended by a hospital surgeon, made of garlic, mustard seed, rad. raphan. balsam of Peru, and gum myrrh using a common drink, barley water well assimilated with tamarinds; by a decoction of which, with the addition of cream of tartar, they were gently purged 3 or 4 times during the course. . . . The consequence was that the most sudden and visible good effects were perceived from the use of oranges and lemons; one of those who had taken them being at the end of 6 days fit for duty.

The results of Lind's work led to the virtual eradication of scurvy at sea. Thus, British sailors became known as "Limeys" because of their daily ration of citrus fruits. It seems likely that many of the nostrums that we now commonly employ in the treatment of the irritable gut will someday be looked upon with the same amazement and disdain with which we regard elixir vitriol, sea water, and vinegar for the treatment of scurvy. Note also Lind's emphasis that the patients all had similar disease, surroundings, and diet, with only the treatments varying among the six pairs.

With several refinements, the controlled clinical trial is in common use today in all fields of medicine. Treatments become blinded, so that the patient does not know what he is receiving and therefore cannot bias the results. This blinding is usually achieved by the use of a placebo pill outwardly identical to the active drug, by a diet induced by intragastric tube, or even in some cases by a sham operation complete with incision. The research physician can also be biased. His enthusiasm for a treatment must be controlled so that studies become double-blinded; that is, only a third party knows which treatment the subject receives. Thus, the observers' assessment of improvement becomes free of bias. It is also considered more statistically valid if the patient acts as his own control. Thus, some trials have a "crossover" design in which the subject receives first one and then the other treatment in random order. This design is best employed in the study of static conditions, such as hypertension, in which subtle differences in blood pressure can be measured against the untreated state. Crossover is less effective in gut reactions, which tend to fluctuate.

Although double-blind, placebo-controlled, possibly crossover clinical trials are a vital instrument to validate the efficacy of treatments new and old, they remain flawed, and the results sometimes fly in the face of common sense. But before we consider the shortcomings of clinical trials in the irritable gut, we need to discuss what is meant by placebo.

PLACEBOS

A Principal Quality of a Physician, as well as a Poet (for Apollo is the God of Physic and Poetry), is of fine lying, or flattering the Patient . . . and it is doubtless as well for the Patient to be Cured by the Working of his Imagination or a Reliance on the Promise of his Doctor, as by repeated Doses of Physic.

P. Shaw (1750)

Thomas Jefferson called placebo pills a "pious fraud." The traditional view has been that some deception is necessary if sugar pills are to be of benefit to the patient. This white lie is justified by many physicians who employ placebos: the end justifies the means. It is now clear that the placebo response is much more complex than traditionally thought, and that it plays a role in almost every therapeutic encounter. Whenever a supposedly inert material is given in an experimental situation, 30 to 60 percent of recipients seem to benefit. In this brief discussion, we will touch upon the impact, nature, and ethics of placebos. For an in-depth analysis, refer to the "Lie That Heals: The Ethics of Giving Placebos," an article by Howard Brody.

Sugar pills or other harmless remedies have been knowingly used by physicians for many generations. It was commonly believed that they often worked, and that patients seemed unsatisfied if they were given nothing. With this need to take something so deeply ingrained in our culture, it could be reasoned that if sugar pills are harmless, and if they work, why not use them? However, the deception and paternalism implied by this traditional approach raise ethical issues. Furthermore, a closer look at these agents has shown us that they have measurable effects that can be achieved without deception.

When placebos are given for pain, narcoticlike substances known as *endorphins* are released by the body and have a pain-relieving effect. This pain relief by placebos may be inhibited by a morphine antagonist drug called naloxone. Furthermore, in clinical trials, patients who are warned of possible side effects of the active drug report experiencing them with the placebo. To demonstrate some of these nonpharmacological effects to medical students, one class was enrolled in the following experiment. The class was divided into 4 groups, with each receiving 1 or 2 of either pink or blue pills. All subjects were conditioned beforehand to expect stimulant or sedative effects. Thirty percent noted changes from these inert pills. The blue pills sedated and the pink pills excited, and two pills had a greater effect than one.

This observation was not an accident: It is known in the pharmaceutical industry that yellow pills are best for depression and green ones for anxiety. Some people develop drug dependence or addiction to placebos. Clearly, the mind–body interaction is important in the placebo response.

We should recognize that the placebo effect plays a role in every therapeutic encounter, and that medicine works best when provided by a caring physician. Even in operations in which a normal organ is removed there may be a happy result. Furthermore, it is held by some individuals that psychotherapy is an elaborate and expensive placebo. In the therapy of the irritable gut, these facts need to be kept in focus. Dyspepsia, the IBS, and other dysfunctions are, after all, benign, long-term illnesses of no mortal consequence. Therefore, is it not more logical to treat them with care, explanation, and reassurance, thus maximizing the placebo response, rather than to prescribe an unproven medication with systemic effects? This may be difficult to do, for people seem conditioned to expect a cure for all ills in a medicine, and to neglect prevention and healthy life style in favor of a therapeutic quick fix. Further implications of the placebo response are discussed next.

PITFALLS OF CLINICAL TRIALS

A cure for functional gut symptoms has been a pharmaceutical imperative for half a century. The notion that one third of the population suffers such symptoms must put a gleam in a marketing executive's eye. Yet, in spite of hundreds of clinical trials, no agent, not even bran, has been convincingly found to be beneficial in the universe of IBS or nonulcer dyspepsia patients, although a few drugs might be employed in special circumstances. We seem to have progressed little from an 1859 therapeutic approach to the IBS that included a trial of therapy of astringents, purgatives, tonics, and mercury.

Few IBS or dyspepsia drug trials are satisfactory by any modern standard. Pitfalls encountered by investigators fall into several categories: faulty hypotheses, unstated or unstratified entry criteria, inappropriate time frame, improper conduct or design, bad statistics, inappropriate extrapolation of results, and neglect of the placebo response.

Faulty Hypotheses

Faulty hypotheses abound. When evaluating a clinical study, we need to ask ourselves whether the question to be answered is sensible. Why should anyone dream that the H_2 blocker cimetidine would be effective in the IBS, or, for that matter, the sedative meprobamate, the opiate antagonists, the beta blockers, the dopamine blockers, or the calcium channel blockers? Even a positive result would not satisfy common sense yet all the above have been tested in clinical trials. There is no generally agreed upon physiologic defect in the IBS, and a shotgun attack on gut chemical receptors is illogical. Such trials might accidentally stumble upon a new pathophysiologic truth; but none have so far.

Unstated Entry Criteria

In a majority of studies, the entry criteria are not stated, or they are so permissive that we cannot be sure what symptoms are being addressed. Since there is no pathophysiologic marker of the various gut reactions, they can be defined only by their symptoms; hence, the need for stratification into symptom groups. The symptoms of those patients who are studied should be clearly stated. It may make sense to use specific drugs to combat diarrhea, constipation, or other specific gut reactions, but a drug of proven benefit for diarrhea cannot be expected to be useful in all IBS patients.

Inappropriate Time Frame

We have seen that the IBS and dyspepsia are chronic relapsing disorders often beginning in youth and lasting a lifetime. Most sufferers do not even seek medical attention. Only one IBS study has extended beyond 6 weeks; one trial was as short as 3 days. It is difficult to reconcile these facts with the use of potent, expensive, systemic drugs administered perhaps over many years, for a benign condition. Should we even be seeking a drug treatment for the irritable gut?

Improper Conduct or Design of the Trial

Klein has reviewed the published IBS treatment trials. He rejected 50 studies because they did not deal exclusively with the IBS under normal living conditions, or because they were not randomized and double-blinded. He analyzed 43 other studies in detail and concluded that "not a single study has been published that provides compelling evidence that any therapeutic agent is efficacious in the global treatment of IBS." The same could be said for most trials of other functional disorders.

Klein also pointed out that many trials are not properly randomized; that is, that the treatment groups are not exactly the same. Demographic factors, such as the sex ratio, may not be the same as those found in society. Crossover studies in which each patient receives both treatments in sequence are not appropriate for a fluctuating condition like the IBS, and yet this design was employed in more than one half of the trials. Too many dropouts made some studies invalid. Thus, the perfect IBS drug trial seems impossible, and we need better methods to test the efficacy of treatment. Klein concluded that "until data to the contrary appear, the scrupulous physician (and patient) would do best to avoid prescribing unproven agents to treat the IBS. Such treatments may result in needless side effects and expense."

Lies, Damn Lies, and Statistics

A detailed discussion of statistical methods is inappropriate, but even those who are untrained in statistics will recognize and understand the flaws pointed out here. Most studies that do not have a control group should not be considered further. Since there is no "gold standard" in the treatment of IBS or dyspepsia, studies that compare one drug with another without placebo are useless.

Further, most studies are very small. Frequently, many questions are asked, thus increasing the possibility of a chance positive result. For example, if 10 criteria are measured before and after treatment, there is a 40 percent likelihood of a positive response to one of them by chance alone. Stratification of patients into conditions, such as diarrhea, constipation, and so on, is often done after the study rather than before—a process that can lend itself to bias. All IBS symptoms are subjective, so how can the physician make a "global assessment" of improvement? A patient may feel better when a tranquilizer is used, but does that tell the physician anything about its effect on the irritable gut? Also, there is a publication bias; negative trials tend not to reach the public eye. This fact and variable, imprecise entry criteria make summary analysis of existing trials useless.

Inappropriate Extrapolation of Results

There is a natural tendency to extrapolate results of a study to conditions beyond that which is tested. Perhaps the best example is the widespread use of cimetidine for nonulcer dyspepsia, a condition that is apparently unrelated to gastric acid levels, whereas the proven benefit of the drug is in acid peptic disease (peptic ulcer).

The Placebo Response

Finally, it is pertinent to discuss the importance of the placebo response in therapeutic trials. Table 31 lists studies of several of the many agents that are used in the treatment of the IBS and dyspepsia. Whether or not the quoted trials show a benefit for a substance in the IBS is irrelevant. It is important, however, to note that the placebo response ranges from 30 to 70 percent. This high placebo response is so consistent in all studies of functional disease that a lower one should make the study suspect. Similar placebo responses are found in clinical trials of some organic diseases, such

Table 31
Placebo Response in Therapeutic Trials

Trials	Drug tested	Percentage of patients with placebo response
Irritable bowel syndrome		
Lichstein, 1969	Belladonna	30
Kasich, 1969	Meprobamate	47
Wayne, 1969	Librax	38
Soltoft, 1975	Bran	65
Fielding, 1982	Domperidone	57
Dyspepsia		
Kolbaek, 1985	Cimetidine and pirenzipine	62
Lance, 1986	Cimetidine	54
Rosch, 1986	Cisapride	28
Nyren, 1986	Antacid and Cimetidine	25

as peptic ulcer. Thus, there are four important lessons to be drawn from these responses. First, placebo responses support the contention that no pharmacotherapy is acceptable for the majority of irritable gut patients without convincing demonstration of efficacy in placebo-controlled, double-blind clinical trials. Second, a trial of therapy is of no value in diagnosis. Note again that peptic ulcer and dyspepsia each have a beneficial response to placebo in up to 50 percent of cases. What diagnostic conclusion can the physician arrive at if a dyspeptic patient improves on an antiulcer drug?

Third, placebos may be useful in certain instances. Some deception is implied by the use of a deliberate or pure placebo, such as a sugar pill. It is said that if a *pure placebo* is to work, the patient should believe that it will have a pharmacologic effect. This may not be entirely true, because clinical trials demand informed consent, yet placebos are still effective. In a small number of neurotic patients, a placebo was effective when the patients knew the pills they were being given were inert. It would seem, therefore, that the symbolic giving of pills has a therapeutic value.

The use of *impure placebos*, that is, drugs whose IBS benefit is not due to the known pharmacology of the drug, risks double deception if both patient and physician come to believe in their efficacy. Nonetheless, certain "impure" or "logical" placebos that have a plausible pharmacologic rationale, yet do no harm, may be useful in certain instances. These might include bran for the IBS, small doses of antacids for dyspepsia, or simethicone for burbulence.

The fourth and probably the most important implication of the placebo response is that it reminds us again of the beneficial effect of the successful physician–patient encounter. "A clinical approach that makes the illness experience more understandable to the patient, that instills a sense of care and social support, and that will increase the feeling of mastery and control over the course of the illness, will be most likely to create a positive placebo response and to improve symptoms." For example, patients who received preoperative explanation of incisional pain, reassurance that medication was available if needed, and pain-avoidance instruction required less medication during their hospital stay than controls. Such a physician–patient interaction involves no deception and is indispensable in the management of the irritable gut. Under ordinary circumstances, no drug need be dispensed. Careful consideration of the patient's complaints, an explanation, and reassurance will be beneficial to many patients.

CONCLUSION

The desire to take medicine appears to be as old as the profession itself. In the chronic, benign, and fluctuating syndromes of the irritable gut, no treatment should be deemed valid without long-term, controlled clinical trials. Unfortunately, such trials are exceedingly difficult, and none, thus far, seem valid for the generality of gut reactions. Because placebos appear to have profound physiologic effects, many sufferers of the irritable gut, and of most other disorders, notice improvement with their use. The implications are that drug treatments for the various gut reactions should not be accepted without properly conducted trials, that response to a certain therapy should not be used as a method of diagnosis, that placebos may be useful in some circumstances, and finally that the successful physician–patient encounter has beneficial effects. At the present time, the best policy is not to employ drugs in the management of the irritable gut except in special circumstances. Perhaps for most gut reactions, no generally effective drug will be found.

CHAPTER TWENTY-TWO

Testing the Irritable Gut

Since by definition the irritable gut has no known pathophysiology, there is no x-ray, blood test, or other measurement that will reliably confirm any of its various syndromes. As repeatedly emphasized, the medical and social history is the principal, indeed, the only instrument of diagnosis. A physical examination provides valuable backup, as physical abnormalities may indicate other disease.

Thus, a test is done to reassure the physician and the patient that no organic condition coexists. Depending upon circumstances, such as the age and sex of the patient, geographic location, family history, and so on, additional testing may be required in some individuals, but common sense should always prevail. Not only are tests expensive, they can sometimes be harmful. They may produce results that contradict all other evidence and, if repeatedly and mindlessly done, may undermine the patient's confidence in his benign diagnosis. A positive diagnosis is the cornerstone of successful management of the irritable gut.

In this chapter, we will describe briefly the tests that patients with the irritable gut must typically undergo. Their indications have been discussed in previous chapters. Only the commonly performed tests are discussed here. An understanding of the principles and methods of testing may make them seem less

329

awesome to us and improve our confidence in their ability to exclude organic disease.

ENDOSCOPY

Fiberoptic technology as applied to endoscopy was invented by the British, developed by the Americans, and marketed by the Japanese; therefore, it is a typical model of international technological development. The operation of the endoscope may be likened to the viewing of a water fountain, in which light from the base of the fountain may be seen to follow a stream of water through its arc. A single glass fiber has the same property so that the light that enters the fiber at one end follows the fiber through bends and loops to exit at the other end. By arranging many fine glass fibers so that their relationship to each other is identical at both ends, it is possible to transmit an image through the bundle. Thus, a gastroscope, which transmits light through its length into the duodenum by one fiber bundle, may transmit the image of the lining of the duodenum back through another bundle around the many twists and turns of the stomach and esophagus to the examiner's eye.

Modern endoscopes are equipped with cables that are controlled by dials that move the tip of the scope to the required attitude. Within the instrument, there is at least one tube through which intestinal juices may be suctioned or through which biopsy forceps, cautery, and other devices may be deployed. Not only are these instruments useful in diagnosis, but there is an increasing number of endoscopic operations that may be done, such as biopsy, cautery of a bleeding lesion, polyp removal, or foreign body retrieval. Not yet in general use are instruments that project images to TV monitors and provide video recordings.

Esophagogastroduodenoscopy (EGD)

A gastroscope is shown in Figure 30. The device to which it is attached contains the external light source and provides suction

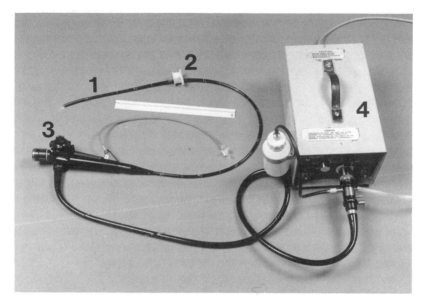

Figure 30. Fiberoptic esophagogastroduodenoscope (EGD). Scope (1) is attached to a device (4) that generates illumination, suction, air pressure to inflate the stomach and, in some cases, electrocautery. Tip of the scope is directed by control knobs (3), and the delicate fiber bundle is protected by a mouthpiece (2) inserted between the teeth. The ruler is 33 centimeters (13½ inches) in length.

and air pressure. The shaft is little more than a meter in length with a diameter similar to that of a pencil. The instrument, on the whole, is quite flexible and light.

A patient undergoing EGD must be fasting (at least 8 hours). Otherwise healthy outpatients usually require no sedation. In our unit, 90 percent of outpatients undergoing this test receive no medication other than a local anesthetic spray to the throat (Xylocaine). This routine avoids the risks attached to drug use, allows full comprehension of the findings by the patient, and permits the patient to return to work soon afterward. Some anxious patients are treated with intravenous diazepam (Valium) or sublingual oxazepam. There is no justification for exposing patients to the risks of a gen-

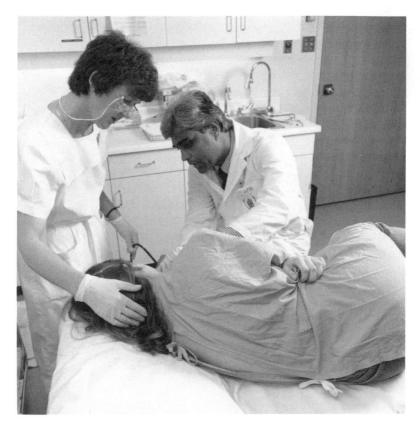

Figure 31. Upper gastrointestinal endoscopy (EGD). With the patient correctly positioned, the endoscopist is introducing the gastroscope with the assistance of a nurse.

eral anesthetic for this procedure. In a series of over 200,000 EGD procedures, the complications of perforation, bleeding, infection, or cardiac events was 0.13 percent, which included patients who were very ill. If the procedure is done by a trained endoscopist in an otherwise healthy patient, the risk is virtually zero.

The patient who is to be examined must be on his left side with his chin toward his chest (Figure 31). After a treatment consent is signed and the local anesthetic spray is applied, the physician gently places his fingers in the patient's throat in order to test that the spray has suppressed gagging, and to familiarize the patient with the sensation of something foreign in the anesthetized throat. It is important to remember that one may breathe normally throughout, since the airway is not obstructed. Saliva should be allowed to drain into a provided towel. A nurse assistant usually urges the patient to breathe because this helps to suppress the gag reflex. The instrument is then placed in the proper position in the throat and the patient is asked to swallow. It is difficult to swallow under these circumstances, but the attempt is usually sufficient to relax the upper esophageal sphincter and allow the instrument to pass into the esophagus. Next, a mouthpiece is placed between the teeth to protect the delicate instrument.

Once the tube is in place, the test lasts approximately 5 minutes. The examination may seem longer to the patient and is certainly not comfortable, but there is usually no pain. Usually, the physician must inject air into the stomach in order to inflate it for better visibility. Before withdrawing the instrument, he may remove most of the air. In some patients, it may be necessary to take a biopsy of the stomach or duodenum, using forceps delivered through the instrument's channel. This additional procedure prolongs the examination a little but it, too, is painless.

When the test is completed, if no sedation is given, the physician can explain the findings and discuss how they will be managed. Of course, in nonulcer dyspepsia, there will be no findings. Nevertheless, the procedure should reassure the patient that no ulcer or other lesion is present in the upper gastrointestinal tract and that therefore no drugs are indicated.

Fibersigmoidoscopy

The fibersigmoidoscope is shown in Figure 32. Similar to the gastroscope, it is about 80 centimeters in length and is structurally thicker to allow more suction capability. Usually, the patient should take a phosphate enema or similar evacuant 2 hours before

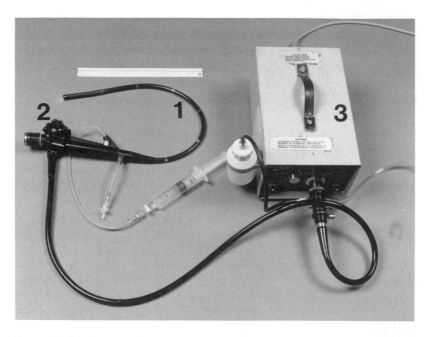

Figure 32. The fibersigmoidoscope (1) is shorter and thicker than the gastroscope. Note controls (2) and light source (3).

the procedure (Chapter 19). No sedation or other preparation is necessary. In cases of severe diarrhea, the enema may be waived.

Once again, the procedure is performed with the patient on his left side, with knees drawn up and feet thrust forward (Figure 33). The physician inspects the area around the patient's anus for fissures, fistulas, hemorrhoids, or other perianal disease and then gently inserts his index finger into the rectum. The purpose of this is to lubricate the canal, to ensure that there is not a lot of feces present, and to exclude any obstructing mass. If there is a painful anal fissure (tiny tear), a local anesthetic lubricant will help a little.

With the assistance of a nurse, the instrument is inserted into the rectum and then maneuvered to its full extent, which is usually just short of the splenic flexure (see Figure 7). At this time, the

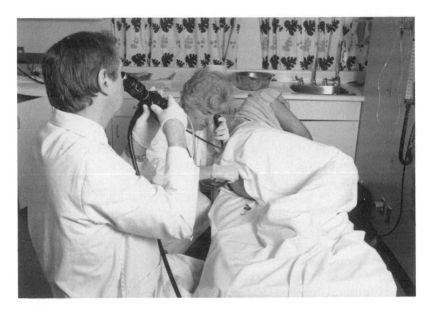

Figure 33. Fibersigmoidoscopy. The endoscopy nurse advances the instrument while the endoscopist uses the controls. Both are able to view the colon.

patient may be seized by an urgent need to defecate or pass gas, but this sensation is just a result of the presence of the instrument. Because the sigmoid colon is somewhat tortuous (sigmoid means S-shaped), the principal difficulty of the procedure is to maneuver around it. Usually, however, the test is accomplished in about 5 minutes. Patients with the irritable bowel syndrome (IBS) may have their pain reproduced by this test, confirming its origin in the colon. Most patients do have some discomfort or pain that is due to looping of the instrument within the sigmoid, but the pain ceases when the instrument is withdrawn. Biopsy may also be done in a manner similar to that employed in EGD.

Immediately, the findings should be explained to the patient; of course, in the irritable gut there should be no disease. Even if a tiny polyp is found, it does not necessarily explain irritable gut symptoms, although it may require removal on its own merits.

Other Endoscopic Procedures

It is possible to examine the entire colon using a *colonoscope*. Usually, a full bowel preparation is necessary as for a barium enema (see below), and sedation is frequently required. Colonoscopy is a lengthier procedure than fibersigmoidoscopy, with more discomfort. In some cases, it may not be possible to maneuver the instrument directly to the cecum. Colonoscopy is not usually indicated for the irritable gut, and the procedure is more costly than sigmoidoscopy plus a barium enema.

Through a side-viewing endoscope placed in the duodenum, a cannula may be passed, which then is threaded into the bile ducts or pancreatic ducts. Contrast material is then injected, which upon x-ray can be seen entering the duct system. This procedure, which is called *endoscopic retrograde-cholangiopancreatography* (ERCP), requires sedation and considerable skill upon the part of the examiner. Serious complications, such as pancreatitis or cholangitis, may result and the test, like colonoscopy, is seldom indicated in the irritable gut. Measuring bile duct pressures through ERCP has been accomplished by some researchers but is not in general use (see Chapter 14).

Enteroscopy (examination of the small bowel) may be performed with a longer endoscope, but for technical reasons, it is difficult to maneuver the instrument beyond the duodenum. Even if successful, the test is too lengthy for practical use.

Rigid Sigmoidoscopy

Although reference to a tube for viewing the rectum appears in the writings of Hippocrates, the first sigmoidoscope was introduced in the late nineteenth century and required candles for illumination. It is fortunate that Thomas Edison invented the light bulb, because colon gas may be explosive (Chapter 12). Until recently, the rigid sigmoidoscope (Figure 34) was the standard test for physicians who wished to examine the rectal mucosa. The instrument is relatively cheap (disposable instruments are now avail-

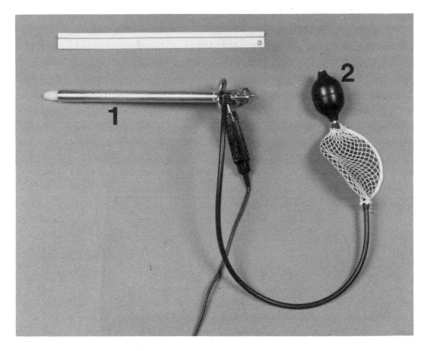

Figure 34. Rigid sigmoidoscope (1). Light is transmitted to the bowel by fiberoptics. The air bulb (2) allows the examiner to distend the rectum for better visibility.

able), and it is easy to clean and use. These features make it very useful in the offices of primary care physicians and surgeons where no fiberoptic equipment exists.

The sigmoidoscopic procedure may be done without any preparation or with a prior Fleet enema. It is easily performed when the patient is in the knee–chest position or on a special sigmoidoscopy table (Figure 35), which permits the bowel to straighten and rectal contents to fall away from the viewer. The rectum can be examined to about 15 centimeters, where it joins the sigmoid usually at a sharp turn. In the majority of cases, the skilled examiner can maneuver the scope around this corner, but the gain in information may not be worth the discomfort. This test is per-

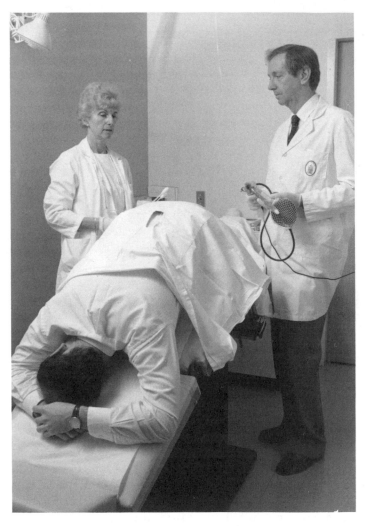

Figure 35. Sigmoidoscopy table permitting the optimum position for a subject undergoing rigid sigmoidoscopy.

fectly acceptable in those patients who have the irritable bowel with no risk factors for organic disease.

BARIUM CONTRAST STUDIES

X-rays, which can blacken photographic film, are able to pass through a human body, casting shadows of bones or other dense structures onto the film. The gut ordinarily casts no shadow, although air in the gut lumen can be recognized as a dark (radiolucent) area and feces can project a mottled appearance. Figure 36 is a "flat film" of the abdomen showing bony structures, gas bubble in the stomach, and gas and feces in the colon. In order to outline the gut, a radio-opaque substance, such as barium, is swallowed or injected via the rectum. X-ray pictures are then taken from various angles to detect any abnormalities of the configuration of the barium within the gut.

Upper Gastrointestinal X-Ray (Esophagus, Stomach, and Duodenum)

By swallowing barium after a fast, the patient renders his esophagus, stomach, and duodenum opaque (Figure 37). The movement of the barium in the gut can be recorded by sequential films, in which a tumor appears as a "filling defect," and an ulcer as a collection of barium in the crater of the ulcer. Properly done, such x-rays detect most ulcers and tumors, but small lesions and esophagitis or gastritis cannot be seen. In the investigation of dyspepsia, this procedure is not the first choice but will do where endoscopy is unavailable or too expensive (Chapter 11). The procedure is also helpful in some cases of noncardiac chest pain or heartburn (Chapters 9 and 10).

Occasionally, it is necessary to examine the small bowel. Often, this examination is required in young patients with diarrhea or chronic abdominal pain in whom Crohn's disease might be suspected; that is, when there is fever, weight loss, bleeding, anemia,

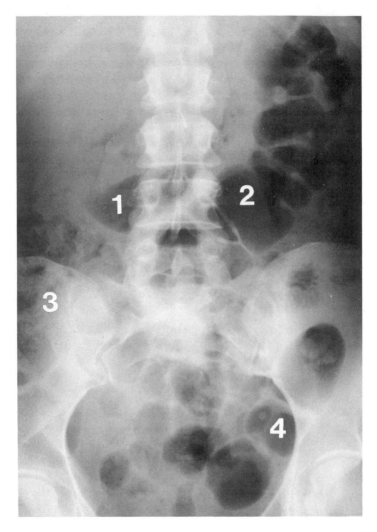

Figure 36. Flat film or plain x-ray of the abdomen showing (1) air in stomach, (2) air in colon (note haustra), (3) air and stool in cecum, and (4) air in sigmoid colon.

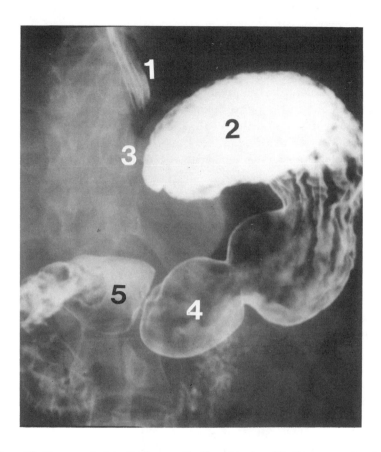

Figure 37. Upper gastrointestinal x-ray. Swallowed barium fills the upper gut and on the x-ray film outlines the esophagus (1), and duodenum (5). Note also the cardia of stomach (2), diaphragm (3), and antrum of stomach (4).

elevated white blood count, or a right lower abdominal mass. Since barium becomes diluted by digestive juices as it makes its way down the gut, it is preferable to insert a tube through the nose and stomach into the duodenum, and to inject the barium in a concentration that renders the entire small bowel opaque, especially the terminal ileum. The tube is uncomfortable, but can be quickly removed. The test is performed more quickly than when the barium is swallowed, and the results are far superior. This procedure is called *enteroclysis* or *small-bowel enema*. A laxative, such as two Dulcolax tablets, is usually taken by the patient the evening before the test.

Barium Enema

For the barium enema procedure to be effective, the colon must be clean (see Figure 26). One of the vigorous preparations that were discussed in Chapter 19 will be required. Each hospital or x-ray department has its own preference, but there are 2 popular techniques. The first is a fluid diet and a magnesium citrate drink given at noon on the day prior to the test, with enemas administered until the return is clear on the day of the test. An increasingly popular method is the colon-washout technique that is accomplished by rapidly drinking 3 to 5 liters of fluid in the few hours preceding the test. The physician ordering the test should provide the patient with detailed instructions.

In the x-ray department, the radiologist inserts a small nozzle into the rectum, and barium flows into the colon under gravity pressure. The modern air contrast technique requires that the excess barium be evacuated once it has coated the bowel wall and air has been injected to highlight mucosal detail. The patient is asked to shift his position on the x-ray table to permit views of the various colon flexures and curves. Properly done, this is a very accurate method of detecting even very small tumors or inflammatory bowel disease.

ULTRASOUND OF THE ABDOMEN

Like x-rays, high-frequency sound waves penetrate the body, casting shadows on a sensitized film or video that signify tissue and structures of varying density. Unlike x-rays, they do not damage tissue. As the technology improves, ultrasound is becoming a popular means by which the abdomen may be examined. In the context of the irritable gut, the ultrasound is useful to exclude gallstones in patients with episodic right upper quadrant abdominal pain, or abdominal masses which might account for pain in the chronic abdomen.

To undergo the test, the patient must be fasting. A lubricated probe is applied to and moved about the abdomen to secure images, as in Figure 38. The procedure is completely painless and harmless.

OTHER TESTS

Blood Tests

A complete blood count (CBC) includes a hemoglobin, white blood cell count, and erythrocyte sedimentation rate. The hemoglobin is the best estimation of the blood's red cell supply. If it is below normal, the patient is said to be anemic. Anemia may have many causes: bleeding, nutritional deficiency, and chronic inflammation, among others, none of which can be due to the irritable gut. An elevated white cell count and sedimentation rate indicate inflammation and these tests should therefore be normal in the irritable gut.

In addition, the physician may choose blood biochemical tests. For example, if serum albumin is low, it may be due to chronic malnutrition or to protein loss from an inflamed gut. Iron, folic acid, and vitamin B_{12} levels may be included if anemia or malabsorption is suspected. Generally, these tests are not done for the irritable gut.

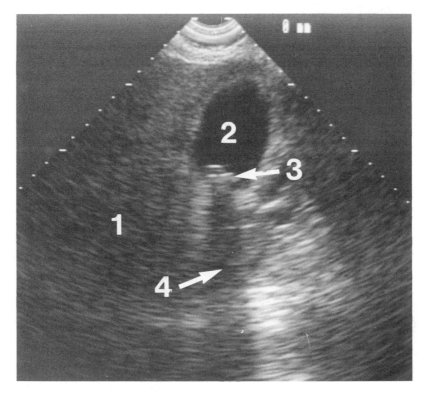

Figure 38. Ultrasound of liver (1) and gallbladder (2). Image shows the fluid-filled gallbladder. A gallstone (3) within the gallbladder blocks the sound waves and casts an *acoustic shadow* (4). This technique is 95 percent to 100 percent accurate in detecting gallstones in the gallbladder.

Tests for Lactose Deficiency

In cases of cramps, gas, and diarrhea, when lactose intolerance is suspect, the physician may do a lactose tolerance test. In this test, 50 grams of lactose is given to a fasting subject in a drink and the blood glucose is measured at intervals thereafter. Failure of blood glucose to rise in response to this drink suggests lactase deficiency and lactose intolerance. An alternative is to measure the breath hydrogen following a lactose drink (Chapter 12). The most important test, however, is the improvement in symptoms when lactose is withdrawn from the diet.

Stool Collections

Occult Blood

Some physicians screen their patients for gut bleeding by asking the patient to provide up to 3 stool specimens, which are analyzed for blood. There are kits available in which a specimen can be applied to a slide and sent to the laboratory by mail. A positive test, particularly if the patient is on a meat-free diet, indicates gastrointestinal bleeding, a phenomenon that is not explained by the irritable gut.

Parasites

The principal parasite of interest in the irritable gut is *Giardia lamblia*. Regrettably, in only 50 percent of cases can their ova be detected by collecting stool. Duodenal specimens obtained by endoscopy are more reliable (Chapter 15). There are a number of other parasites that may be found coincidentally in the irritable gut but that are not recognized as being pathogenetic. Thus, it is important that they not be treated as the cause of gut symptoms.

Stool Collection for Fat

In cases in which malabsorption is suspected, a 3-day stool collection may be very useful. Generally, the patient is placed on an 80-gram fat diet 24 to 48 hours prior to the beginning of the collection. Commencing at 8:00 AM, the stool is collected in a pre-weighed container for 72 hours. All stools (with no urine or toilet paper) must be included. The container is again weighed and the daily weight of its contents calculated. This figure is very useful because if it exceeds 300 to 500 grams per day, an organic cause is likely. The stool may also be analyzed for fat. The fat content is elevated in malabsorption/maldigestion states, such as celiac disease or pancreatic insufficiency. If the stool is liquid, its sodium, potassium, magnesium, and other mineral contents can be measured, and analytic techniques are available for the detection of various laxatives (Chapter 19). It is important that all stool produced in the 72-hour period be collected, and that the container be kept in a cool place and brought promptly to the lab when the collection is done.

SUMMARY

There is no test for the irritable gut. Depending upon the circumstances, a minimal number of tests may be required to firmly exclude organic disease and to achieve confidence in a functional one. The tests described here are relatively safe and usually only one or two are necessary. For example, sigmoidoscopy is important in the irritable bowel syndrome, and a barium enema may be added if the patient is over 40 years of age. An endoscopy is an essential means by which nonulcer dyspepsia is distinguished from peptic ulcer. Further tests, such as enteroclysis, CAT scan, ERCP, kidney x-rays, and stool collection should be reserved for specific suspicions.

Epilogue

We have come to the end of our journey through the often troubled gut. By now you should know enough about gut reactions to view skeptically anybody who claims that the causes or the cures are known. You should realize that there are many schools of thought on the irritable gut, including those which believe it is psychogenic. Depression, anxiety, or other psychological states might cause the symptoms, might result from the symptoms, or might even impair one's ability to cope with the symptoms. Other medical authorities believe the cause is dietary, perhaps a lack of dietary fiber. Still others remain convinced that the irritable gut is caused by a physiologic defect for which a correcting drug will someday be found. But can diarrhea, constipation, globus, or dyspepsia be caused by a single defect? Thoughtful researchers like Thomas Almy wonder if gut reactions are abnormal at all. Are they a disease for which a cure should be sought, or are they rather the way in which the gut responds to its owner's psychosocial and dietary environment? All these viewpoints merit serious consideration.

You should also believe that these symptoms are real and often not trivial. Yet they are neither mortal nor physically disabling. Although they may be difficult to eradicate, you should not permit gut reactions to interfere with your life. A lifelong search for a cure may be doomed to failure, but, clearly, there are some common-sense changes in life-style that may ease the symptoms. In some cases, dietary fiber may help. Alcohol, tobacco, and improper eating habits can be forsworn. Recognize also that life's stresses may aggravate or precipate some gut reactions. Regular exercise is often helpful, but only if it brings enjoyment.

Whatever the cause (or causes) of the irritable gut eventually turns out to be, the sensible approach, at least at this time, is to be reassured that no structural disease exists, to make appropriate changes in your life-style, and to avoid tests, drugs, or nostrums that may, in the end, do more harm than the symptoms they are supposed to cure.

Bibliography

CHAPTER 2

Connell AM: Intestinal motility and the irritable bowel. *Postgrad Med* 1984;60:791–796.

Sarna SK: Motor correlates of functional gastrointestinal symptoms. *Viewpoints on Digestive Dis* 1988;20:1.

Thompson WG: Gut motility, in Thompson WG: *The Irritable Gut*. Baltimore, University Park Press, 1979, Chap 1.

CHAPTER 3

Cummings JH, Jenkins DJA, Wiggens HS: Measurement of the mean transit time of dietary residue through the gut. *Gut* 1976;17:210–218.

Drossman DA, Sandler RS, McKee DC, Lovitz AJ: Bowel dysfunction among subjects not seeking health care. *Gastroenterology* 1982;83:529–534.

Thompson WG: *The Irritable Gut*. Baltimore, University Park Press, 1979, Chap 2.

Thompson WG, Heaton KW: Functional bowel disorder in apparently healthy people. *Gastroenterology* 1980;79:283–288.

CHAPTER 4

Thompson WG, Heaton KW: Functional gastrointestinal disorders in apparently healthy people. *Gastroenterology* 1980;79:283–288.

Thompson WG, Drossman DA, Heaton KW, Kruis W, Doteval G: Working Team Report: Guidelines for the diagnosis of the irritable bowel. Proceedings of 13th International Congress of Gastroenterology. Rome, Italy September 1988. *Gastroenterology Int* 1989;92–96.

CHAPTER 5

Almy T: The irritable bowel syndrome: Back to square one? *Dig Dis Sci* 1980;25:401–403.
Drossman DA, Sandler RS, McKee DC, Lovitz DJ: Bowel dysfunction among subjects not seeking health care. *Gastroenterology* 1982;83:529–534.
Thompson WG: Irritable bowel syndrome: Prevalence, prognosis and consequences. *Can Med J* 1986;134:111–113.
Whitehead WE, Winget C, Fedaravicius AS, *et al*: Learned illness behavior in subjects with irritable bowel syndrome and peptic ulcer. *Dig Dis Sci* 1982;27:202–208.

CHAPTER 6

Burkitt DP, Walker ARP, Painter NS: Effect of dietary fiber on stools and transit times, and its role in the causation of disease. *Lancet* 1972;2:1408–1411.
Cleave TL: *The Saccharine Disease*. Bristol, England, Wright & Sons Ltd, 1974.
Cummings JH: Dietary fiber. *Br Med Bull* 1981;37:65–70.
Eastwood MA, Passmore R: Dietary fiber. *Lancet* 1983;2:202–206.
Marcus SN, Heaton KW: Deoxycholic acid and the pathogenesis of gallstones. *Gut* 1988;29:522–533.
McCance RA, Widdowson WM: Old thoughts and new work on bread white and brown. *Lancet* 1955;2:205–210.
Ornstein MH, Baird IM: Dietary fiber and the colon. *Mol Aspects Med* 1987;9:41–67.
Thompson WG: Dietary fiber, in Thompson WG: *The Irritable Gut*. Baltimore, University Park Press, 1979, pp 27–40.

CHAPTER 7

Almy TP, Abbott FK, Hinkle LE: Alteration in colonic function under stress. *Gastroenterology* 1950;15:95–103.
Creed F, Guthrie E: Psychological factors in the irritable bowel syndrome. *Gut* 1987;28:1307–1318.

Drossman DA: The physician and the patient, in Sleisinger M, Fortran J: *Diseases of the Gastrointestinal Tract*. Philadelphia, Saunders, 1983, pp 1–19.

Drossman DA, McKee DL, Sandler RS, et al: Psychosocial factors in the irritable bowel syndrome: A multivariate study of patients and non-patients with irritable bowel syndrome. *Gastroenterology* 1988;95:701–708.

Engel GL: Psychogenic pain and the pain-prone patient. *Am J Med* 1959;26:899–918.

Latimer PR: *Functional Gastrointestinal Disorders: A Behavioural Medicine Approach*. New York, Springer, 1983.

Mansour RA, Smith GR: Somatization disorders in primary care. *New Engl J Med* 1983;308:1464–1465.

McRae S, Younger K, Thompson DG, Wingate DL: Sustained mental stress alters human jejunal motor activity. *Gut* 1982;23:404–409.

Thompson WG: Gut reaction, in Thompson WG: *The Irritable Gut*. Baltimore, University Park Press, 1979, pp 41–48.

Whitehead WE, Bosmajian L, Zonderman AB, et al: Symptoms of psychologic distress associated with irritable bowel syndrome. Comparison of community and medical clinic samples. *Gastroenterology* 1988;95:709–720.

CHAPTER 8

Glaser JP, Engel GL: Psychodynamics, psychophysiology, and gastrointestinal symptomatology. *Clin Gastroenterology* 1977;6:507–531.

Palmer ED: *Functional Gastrointestinal Disease*. Baltimore, Williams and Wilkins, 1967.

Thompson WG: Globus, in Thompson WG: *The Irritable Gut*. Baltimore, University Park Press, 1979, Chap 16.

Thompson WG, Heaton KW: Heartburn and globus in apparently healthy people. *Can Med Assoc J* 1982;126:46–48.

CHAPTER 9

Clouse RE, Lustman PJ: Psychiatric illness and contraction abnormalities of the esophagus. *New Engl J Med* 1983;309:1337–1342.

Peters L, Mass L, Petty D, et al: Spontaneous non-cardiac chest pain evaluation by 24 hour ambulatory esophageal motility and pH monitoring. *Gastroenterology* 1988;94:977–983.

Richter JE, Castell DO: Esophageal disease as a cause of noncardiac chest pain. *Adv Intern Med* 1988;33:311–336.

Richter JE, Bradley LA, Castell DO: Esophageal chest pain: Current controversies in pathogenesis, diagnosis and therapy. *Ann Intern Med* 1989;110:66–78.

Vantrappen G, Janssens J: What is irritable esophagus: Another point of view. *Gastroenterology* 1988;94:1092–1093.

CHAPTER 10

Burkitt DP, James PA: Low residue diets and hiatus hernia. *Lancet* 1973;2:128–130.

Castell DO: Medical therapy for reflux esophagitis: 1986 and beyond. *Ann Intern Med* 1986;104:112–114.

MacCara ME, Nugent FJ, Garner JB: Acid neutralization capacity of Canadian antacid formulations. *Can Med Assoc J* 1985;132:523–527.

Thompson WG: Heartburn, in Thompson WG: *The Irritable Gut*. Baltimore, University Park Press, 1979, Chap 12.

Thompson WG, Heaton KW: Heartburn and globus in apparently healthy people. *Can Med Assoc J* 1982;126:46–48.

CHAPTER 11

Beaumont W: Experiments and observations on the gastric juice and the physiology of digestion (facsimile of 1833 edition), New York, Dover, 1959, p 107.

Nyren O, Adani HO, Gustevsson S, *et al*: The "epigastric distress syndrome" :A possible disease entity identified by history and endoscopy in patients with non-ulcer dyspepsia. *J Clin Gastroenterol* 1987;9:303–309.

Talley NJ, Phillips SF: Non-ulcer dyspepsia potential cause and pathophysiology. *Ann Int Med* 1988;108:865–879.

Thompson WG: Non-ulcer dyspepsia. *Can Med Assoc J* 1984;130:565–569.

Thompson WG: Psychogenic vomiting, in Thompson WG: *The Irritable Gut*. Baltimore, University Park Press, 1979, Chap 15.

CHAPTER 12

Fardy J, Sullivan S: Gastrointestinal gas. *Can Med Assoc J* 1988;139:1137–1142.

Kantor, JL. A study of atmospheric air in the upper digestive tract. *Amer J Med Sci* 1918:155;820–856.

Levitt MD: Intestinal gas production—recent advances in flatology. *New Engl J Med* 1980;302:1474–1475.

Levitt MD, Bond JH: Intestinal gas, Sleisenger M, Fortran J (eds): *Gastrointestinal Disease*, ed 3. Philadelphia, Saunders, 1983, pp 222–227.

Thompson, WG. Burbulence, in Thompson WG: *The Irritable Gut*. Baltimore, University Park Press, 1979, Chap 13.

Thompson, WG: Burbulence (Indigestion due to gas). *Can Med Assoc J* 1972;106:1220–1225.

CHAPTER 13

Almy TP: The irritable bowel syndrome: Back to square one? *Dig Dis Sci* 1980;25:401–403.
Chaudhary NA, Truelove SC: The irritable colon syndrome. *Q J Med* 1962;31:307–323.
Kruis W, Thieme CH, Weinzierl M, *et al*: A diagnostic score for the irritable bowel syndrome: its value in the exclusion of organic disease. *Gastroenterology* 1984;87:1–7.
Manning AP, Thompson WG, Heaton KW, Morris AF: Towards positive diagnosis of the irritable bowel. *Br Med J* 1978;2:653–654.
McRae S, Younger K, Thompson DG, Wingate DL: Sustained mental stress alters human jejunal motor activity. *Gut* 1982;23:404–409.
Southgate DAT, Bailey B, Collinson E, Walker AF: A guide to calculating intakes of dietary fibre. *J Clin Nutr* 1976;30:303–310.
Svedlund J, Sjoden L, Ottoson JO, Dotexall G: Controlled study of psychotherapy in irritable bowel syndrome. *Lancet* 1983;2:589–691.
Swarbrick ET, Hegarty JE, Bat L, *et al*: Site of pain from the irritable bowel. *Lancet* 1980;2:443–446.
Thompson WG, Dotevall G, Drossman DA, Heaton KW, Kruis W: The irritable bowel: Guidelines for the diagnosis. *Gastroenterology Int* 1989;2:92–96.
Thompson WG: The irritable bowel. *Gut* 1984;25:305–320.
Thompson WG: A strategy for management of the irritable bowel. *Am J Gastroenterol* 1986;81:95–100.
Thompson WG: The irritable bowel syndrome, in Phillips, SF: *The Large Intestine: Physiology, Pathophysiology and Diseases*. Saunders, 1990, Chap 25. (in press)
Wright SH, Snape WJ, Battle W, *et al*: Effect of dietary components on gastrocolonic response. *Amer J Physiology* 1980;238:228–232.

CHAPTER 14

Alexander-Williams J: Do adhesions cause pain? *Br Med J* 1987;294:659–660.
Asher R: Münchhausen syndrome. *Lancet* 1951;1:339–341.
Creed F: Life events and appendectomy. *Lancet* 1981;1:1381–1385.
Engel GL: Psychogenic pain and the pain-prone patient. *Am J Med* 1959;26:899–918.
Heaton KW: Pelvic pain in women. *Br Med J* 1986;293:1504.
Hutcheson R: The chronic abdomen. *Br Med J* 1923;1:667–669.
Kingham JGC, Dawson AM: Origin of chronic right upper quadrant pain. *Gut* 1985;26:737–738.
Pfeiffer E: Treating the patient with confirmed functional pain. *Hosp Phys* 1971;6:68–72.

Thompson WG: The chronic abdomen, in Barkin V, Rogers A (eds), *Difficult Decisions in Digestion*. New York, Yearbook, 1988, Chap 10.
Tryer SP: Learned pain behaviour. *Br Med J* 1986;292:1–3.

CHAPTER 15

Read NW (ed): *Diarrhoea: New Insights*. London, Jansen Marlow, 1981.
Thompson WG: Functional diarrhoea, in Thompson WG: *The Irritable Gut*. Baltimore, University Park Press, 1979, Chap 7.

CHAPTER 16

Devroede G, Poisson J, Shang JC: Obstipation: What is the appropriate therapeutic approach? In Barkin J, Rogers AI (eds), *Difficult Decisions in Digestive Diseases*. New York, Yearbook, 1989, pp 458–484.
Gant SG: *Constipation and Intestinal Obstruction*. Philadelphia, WB Saunders, 1909.
Hertz AF: *Constipation and Allied Intestinal Disorders*. London, Oxford University Press, 1909.
Read NW, Timms JM: Pathophysiology of constipation. *Acta Gastroenterol Belg* 1987;50:393–404.
Thompson WG: Constipation, in Thompson WG: *The Irritable Gut*. Baltimore, University Park Press, 1979, pp 93–105.

CHAPTER 17

Barkan MB: Proctalgia fugax. *Klin Med* 1966;44:110–113.
Ibrahim H: Proctalgia fugax. *Gut* 1961;2:137–140.
Myrtle AS: Some common afflictions of the anus often neglected by medical men and patients. *Brit Med J* 1883;1:1061–1062.
Thaysen TEH: Proctalgia fugax. *Lancet* 1935;2:243–246.
Thompson WG: Proctalgia fugax: A review. *Dig Dis Sci* 1981;26:1121–1124.
Thompson WG: Proctalgia fugax in patients with the irritable bowel, peptic ulcer or inflammatory bowel disease. *Am J Gastroenterol* 1984;79:450–452.
Thompson WG, Heaton KW: Proctalgia fugax. *J Roy Coll Phys Lond* 1980;14:247–248.

CHAPTER 18

Almy TP, Howell DA: Diverticular disease of the colon. *N Engl J Med* 1980;302:324–331.

Sim GPG, Scobie BA: Large bowel diseases in New Zealand based on 1118 air contrast enemas. *N. Zealand Med* 1982;95:611–613.

Spriggs EI, Marxor OA: Intestinal diverticula. *Qu J Med* 1925;19:1–34.

Thompson WG, Patel DG: Clinical picture of diverticular disease of the colon. *Clin Gastroenterology* 1986;15:903–916.

Thompson WG, Patel DG, Tao H, Nair RC: Does uncomplicated diverticular disease cause symptoms. *Dig Dis Sci* 1982;27:605–608.

CHAPTER 19

Cummings JH: Laxative abuse. *Gut* 1974;15:158–166.

DiPalma JA, Brandy CE: Comparison of colon cleansing methods in preparation for colonoscopy. *Gastroenterology* 1984;86:856–860.

Morris AI, Turnberg LA: Surreptitious laxative abuse. *Gastroenterology* 1979;77:780–786.

Read NW, Krejg J, Read MG, et al: Chronic diarrhoea of unknown origin. *Gastroenterology* 1980;78:264–271.

Smith S. Cited in: In England now. *Lancet* 1973;2:1079.

Tedesco FJ: Laxative use in constipation. *Am J Gastroenterol* 1985;80:303–309.

Thompson WG: Catharsis, in Thompson WG: *The Irritable Gut*. Baltimore, University Park Press, 1979, pp 107–124.

Witts LJ: Ritual purgation in modern medicine. *Lancet* 1937;1:427–430.

CHAPTER 20

Barone FC, White RF, Ormsbee HS, et al: Effects of calcium channel entry blockers, nifedipine and nilvadipine on colonic motor activity. *J Pharmacol Exp Ther* 1986;237(1):99–106.

Bruks TF: Actions of drugs on gastrointestinal motility, in Johnson LR (ed): *Physiology of the Gastrointestinal Tract*, ed 2. New York, Raven Press, 1987, pp 723–743.

Farrar JT: The effects of drugs on intestinal motility. *Clin Gastroenterology* 1982;11(3):673–681.

Hoffman BB: Adrenergic receptor-activating drugs, in Katzung BG (ed): *Basic and Clinical Pharmacology*, ed 2. Los Altos, California, Lange Medical Publications, 1984, pp 86–106.

Jaffe JH, Martin WR: Opioid analgesics and antagonists, in Gilman AG, Goodman LS, Rall TO (eds): *The Pharmacological Basis of Therapeutics*, ed 7. New York, Macmillan, 1985, pp 491–531.

Jay BH, Abrahamsson H, Stockbruegger RW, et al: Effect of selective and non-selective antimuscarinics on rectosigmoid motility and gastrointestinal transit. *Scand J Gastroenterol* 1985;20:1101–1109.

Lees GM, Percy WH: Antibiotic associated colitis: An in vitro investigation of the effects of antibiotics on intestinal motility. *Br J Pharmacol* 1981;73:553–547.

Khalil MK, Thompson WG: Disorders of intestinal motility resulting from drug therapy, in Snape WJ (ed): *Pathogenesis of Functional Bowel Disease*, New York, Plenum, 1989, Chap 6, pp. 101–112.

Moncada S, Flower JR, Vane JR: Prostaglandins, prostacyclin, thromboxane A and leukotrienes, in Gilman AG, Goodman LS, Rall TW et al (eds): *The Pharmacological Basis of Therapeutics*, ed 7. New York, Macmillan, 1985, p 667.

Schindler JS, Finnerty GJ, Towlson K, et al: Domperidone and levodopa in Parkinson's disease. *Br J Clin Pharmacol* 1984;18:959–962.

VanNueten JM, Schuurkes JAJ: Studies on the role of dopamine and dopamine blockers in gastroduodenal motility. *Scand J Gastroenterol* 1984 [Suppl 96]:90–99.

CHAPTER 21

Brody H: The lie that heals: The ethics of giving placebos. *Ann Intern Med* 1982;97:112–118.

Klein KB: Controlled clinical trials in the irritable bowel syndrome: A critique. *Gastroenterology* 1988;95:232–241.

Lind J: A Treatise of the Scurvey in Stewart CP, Guthrie D (eds): *Lind's Treatise on Scurvey*: Bicentenary Volume. Edinburgh, University Press, 1953.

Nelson RB: Are clinical trials pseudoscience? *Forum in Medicine*, 1979;594–860 (September).

CHAPTER 22

Thompson WG: Sigmoidoscopy, in Thompson WG: *The Irritable Gut*. Baltimore, University Park Press, 1979, p 49.

Thompson WG, Dotevall G, Drossman DA, Heaton KW, Kruis W: The irritable bowel: Guidelines for the diagnosis. *Int J Gastroenterology* 1989;2:

Index